Evidence-Based Interventions
for Children with Challenging Behavior

Kathleen Hague Armstrong
Julia A. Ogg
Ashley N. Sundman-Wheat
Audra St. John Walsh

Evidence-Based Interventions for Children with Challenging Behavior

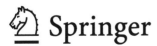 Springer

Kathleen Hague Armstrong
Department of Pediatrics
College of Medicine
University of South Florida
Tampa, FL, USA

Julia A. Ogg
Department of Psychological & Social
  Foundations
University of South Florida
Tampa, FL, USA

Ashley N. Sundman-Wheat
School Psychology
District School Board of Pasco County
Land O'Lakes, FL, USA

Audra St. John Walsh
Department of Pediatrics
College of Medicine
University of South Florida
Tampa, FL, USA

ISBN 978-1-4614-7806-5   ISBN 978-1-4614-7807-2 (eBook)
DOI 10.1007/978-1-4614-7807-2
Springer New York Heidelberg Dordrecht London

Library of Congress Control Number: 2013941039

Printed on acid-free paper

Springer is part of Springer Science+Business Media (www.springer.com)

This book is gratefully dedicated to the children and caregivers who have taught us so much, and to the providers who are committed to ensuring that all children learn and develop to their best potential.

Contents

Chapter 1
Common Early Childhood Behavior Problems

Abstract Challenging behavior in young children is common. It can be difficult for parents or early childhood professionals to know what behaviors fall within the typical range of behavior. This chapter outlines the prevalence of common behavioral concerns among young children (sleep problems, feeding issues, colic/excessive crying, toileting issues, fears/worries/anxiety, sexual behaviors, aggression, and social skills) and outlines guidelines for how to address these concerns. Strategies to ensure cultural competence in working with a diverse range of families are also outlined.

Keywords Behavior problems • Behavior disorder • Sleep problems • Sleep disorders • Sleep hygiene • Feeding problems • Colic • Toilet training • Anxiety • Fear • Worries • Sexual behaviors • Sexual behavior problems • Aggression • Parent–child interaction • Social skills • Autism spectrum disorders • Attention-deficit/hyperactivity disorder • Cultural competence

Behavior problems in young children are common (Williams, Klinepeber, & Palmes, 2004). Healthy toddlers are extremely active, restless, and impulsive, not because they have a disorder, but because they need to move about and experience to learn. Furthermore, each child comes with his or her own temperament, making for huge variations of personalities, even within families. Providing parents with basic parenting guidelines can help most families successfully navigate through the early childhood years. These strategies, such as developing and maintaining consistent routines, removing dangerous temptations, praising desired behavior, and redirecting problem behavior, are beneficial to all children.

Even so, approximately 20 % of US children have a diagnosable behavioral health disorder, and less than 20 % of those in need will receive help (Society for Research in Children's Development, 2009; U.S. Public Health Service, 2001). Upon entering kindergarten, problem behaviors, especially aggression and hyperactivity, place children at risk not only for poor academic outcomes but also for social-emotional and behavioral problems in school which may persist throughout adulthood (Coie & Dodge, 1998; Dishion, French, & Patterson, 1995; Tremblay, 2000). Thus, it becomes important to differentiate between behaviors that are normal and will possibly be outgrown and those needing more individualized attention.

It can be difficult to separate typical behaviors of early childhood from those that would be considered problematic. For example, problems such as sleep difficulties or short attention spans may be typical with young children, but those issues become more problematic as children get older. Research suggests that rather than just considering the behavior by itself, one might want to observe for patterns of behavior (Mathiesen & Sanson, 2000). For example, early onset behavior problems such as aggression and noncompliance are more likely to be indicative of later problems if they are exhibited across settings, including home and daycare, rather than in just one setting (Miller, Koplewicz, & Klein, 1997).

The next sections provide information on a number of common behavioral concerns in early childhood, including sleep problems, feeding issues, colic/excessive crying, toileting issues, fears/worries/anxiety, sexual behaviors, aggression, and social skills. These challenging behaviors were selected for discussion because (1) they are frequent concerns for young children and their families (prevalence rates for most is at least 20 %), (2) they are issues presented frequently in our clinical practice, and (3) these difficulties have been described by other authors as prevalent concerns in young children (e.g., Young, Davis, Schoen, & Parker, 1998). This overview is intended to help early childhood professionals know what behaviors can be expected during the typical course of development, and to be able to distinguish behaviors which may be indicative of more serious and chronic problems in need of more intensive intervention. Information about these common concerns as well as guidelines to promote healthy development are presented.

Sleep Problems

Prevalence

Sleep problems are one of the most commonly reported difficulties in young children, and may be associated with a variety of conditions and medical problems. Sleep is important for renewing mental and physical health, while sleep disorders can lead to reduced health and in some cases may be life threatening (Luginbuehl, Bradley-Klug, Ferron, Anderson, & Benbadis, 2008). Research suggests that between 20 and 25 % of children and adolescents may have a sleep disorder (Mindell, Owens, & Carskadon, 1999), yet few are screened and treated (Luginbuehl et al., 2008). Children with developmental disabilities, asthma, and other medical conditions are at increased risk for sleep problems (Armstrong, Kohler, & Lilly, 2009; Buckhalt, Wolfson, & El-Sheikh, 2007). A number of factors have been

Table 1.1 National Sleep Foundation Guidelines for hours of sleep needed

Age	Hours of sleep
Infants (3–11 months)	9–12 h during the night +
	30 min to 2-h naps, 1–4 times a day
Toddlers (1–3 years)	12–14 h
Preschool (3–5 years)	11–13 h
School-aged children (5–12 years)	10–11 h (children typically do not nap after 5 years)

associated with disturbed sleep in young children, including maternal depression, being introduced to solid foods prior to 4 months of age, attending childcare outside of the home, and watching TV/videos (Nevarez, Rifas-Shiman, Kleinman, Gillman, & Taveras, 2010).

The most common sleep problems in young children are difficulty falling asleep, waking up during the night, or a combination of both (Lyons-Ruth, Zeanah, & Benoit, 2003). In addition, toddlers and preschool children may have difficulty with nightmares, night terrors, sleepwalking, and sleep talking (Armstrong, Kohler, & Lilly, 2009).

Guidelines

According to the National Sleep Foundation (http://www.sleepfoundation.org/), by 6 months of age, infants can learn to sleep for at least 9 h per night, and by 9 months 70–80 % of infants are able to sleep through the night. Table 1.1 outlines the National Sleep Foundation Guidelines for the amount of sleep needed by children, and may be used to help parents begin to pinpoint sleep problems and take steps to improve sleep.

To address difficulty falling asleep, the first step is to alter the child's sleep habits, often referred to as sleep hygiene. Sleep hygiene includes strategies which can be used to solve sleep problems and begins with the establishment of a regular nighttime routine. Difficulty falling asleep can be a pattern of behavior which develops because the child has connected the action of falling to sleep with something else, generally related to the parent, such as rocking, being held, nursed, or some sort of motion, and cannot fall asleep by him or herself. To correct this sleep problem, parents have to reteach the child to fall asleep with a new set of associations, such as a blanket or stuffed animal. The process involves developing a relaxing bedtime routine, followed by gradual separation from the child beginning with 2 min intervals, and brief comforting to let child know he or she is safe. Parents will find this intervention difficult to follow because their child will protest, and will need encouragement to stay the course. Most children will learn to sleep on their own within 5 days of consistent teaching (Ferber, 2009).

Even when caregivers are attempting to set healthy routines, limit setting problems around bedtime generally begin around age 2, when toddlers are naturally testing limits, and resolve when parents develop consistent bedtime routines and remain firm in their expectations. Bedtime routines that help children sleep well include wind down activities such as a warm bath; avoidance of television or other media before bed; keeping bedrooms cool, dark, and distraction-free; and building in time for some personal interaction at bedtime, like reading books or saying prayers. Parents should also avoid giving their child food or drinks containing caffeine, or over-the-counter cough medications that contain stimulants.

To address the issue of young children staying asleep during the night, an initial consideration is nighttime feedings. Nighttime feeding problems are addressed by gradually reducing the habit of providing the child with food at night. By 6 months of age, a baby should be able to sleep through the night without feeding or feeling hungry (National Sleep Foundation, 2010). Nursing babies can wait to be fed in increasingly longer intervals, until nighttime feedings are eliminated. Bottle-fed babies are offered one ounce less at each feeding and at less frequent intervals during the night, until the problem is resolved. A protein snack shortly before bed for older children can help ease hunger until morning.

Feeding Issues

Prevalence

Feeding problems are very common, with estimates of prevalence as high as 35 % in young children (Jenkins, Bax, & Hart, 1980). Feeding issues become evident at different stages of infancy and early childhood, with the prevalence of feeding problems increasing with age. Four percent of children at 18 months experience significant feeding problems, while at 30 months this number rises to 8 % (Mathiesen & Sanson, 2000). When moderate feeding problems are considered, 47 % of children at age 18 months are considered by parents to have a problem, while at 30 months, 62 % were considered to have moderate feeding problems (Mathiesen & Sanson, 2000).

On the extreme side of pediatric feeding issues is failure to thrive. Failure to thrive is diagnosed in children whose weight falls below the fifth percentile for age on growth charts (Lyons-Ruth et al., 2003). One to five percent of all pediatric hospital admissions are due to failure to thrive (American Psychiatric Association [*DSM-IV-TR*], 2000), providing evidence of how severe feeding problems can become in young children.

Although there is not clear consensus in the literature, it is believed the feeding problems in young children can result from organic and nonorganic causes. For example, physical difficulty with the feeding process can be one organic reason that children have difficulty getting adequate nutrients through their food. Chronic medical issues such as reflux can make eating very painful and set up an aversion to feedings. Alternatively, some nonorganic feeding problems develop and are maintained by problematic parent–child relationships, expectations, and lack of mealtime routines. For example, children may refuse healthy foods during dinner because they have learned that they will be allowed to have preferred snacks later.

Guidelines

Most professional guidelines, including those from the American Academy of Pediatrics (AAP) and the World Health Organization (WHO), recommend breast milk or formula as the main food for children until 6 months of age. The AAP recommends that solid foods be introduced no sooner than between 4 and 6 months of age. The WHO has reported that the introduction of complementary feeding (or transitioning from breastfeeding or formula to other foods) can be a "vulnerable" time period for young children. The WHO guidelines suggest that complementary feeding should begin around 6 months. They also recommend that the nutritional value of the complementary foods be high and free of possible toxins.

Parents are often concerned with how much food their child should eat, especially once they start to introduce foods that are not premeasured in jars. The United States Department of Agriculture (USDA) recommends the following calorie guidelines for young children each day:

- Around 520–570 calories for children 0–6 months
- Around 676–743 calories for children ages 7–12 months
- Around 992–1,046 calories for children ages 1–2 years
- Around 1,642–1,743 calories for children ages 3–8 years

Beginning at age 2, calories should be obtained from six servings from the Grain food group, three from the Vegetable food group, two from the Fruit group, two from the Milk group, and two from the Meat and Beans Group.

In addition to the guidelines for how much to eat, the AAP also offers tips for dealing with feeding and eating issues:

- Don't threaten, punish, or force-feed your child.
- Provide structure at mealtime with regard to the timing and seating requirements for mealtime. In other words, have mealtimes on a regular schedule and require your child to sit at the table to minimize other distractions.
- Prepare several healthy foods you would be ok with your child eating and allow them to choose which foods they want to eat.
- Limit the length of time for meals.
- Avoid making special meals for children who are picky. Instead, include one preferred item in the meal and encourage the child to try other foods.
- Food refusal should not be rewarded by offering snacks or preferred foods.

Colic/Excessive Crying

Prevalence

Colic and excessive crying are common problems in very young children (from birth to about 6 months old). Colic is often defined by "Wessel's Rule of Threes" which describes colic as:

- Crying for at least 3 h a day
- For at least 3 days in any 1 week
- For at least 3 weeks

This group of symptoms becomes colic when they occur in an otherwise healthy infant and when no cause for the child's discomfort can be identified (Lucassen et al., 1998). Studies of the prevalence of colic have generated estimates as high as 40 % of young children, but most estimates indicate that between 14 and 19 % of families seek assistance from a physician (Lucassen et al., 2001). The prevalence of colic decreases with age, as one study found that up to 29 % of infants between 1 and 3 months had colic, but once a child is between 4 and 6 months old, the prevalence drops to 7–11 % (St. James-Roberts & Halil, 1991). The cause of colic is often unknown and may include painful intestinal contractions, lactose intolerance, food allergies, gas, or have no physical cause at all. In addition, a parent may perceive normal amounts of crying as being in excess (Lucassen et al., 1998).

Guidelines

There are few effective interventions for colic, and most cases resolve without intervention by 6 months of age. However, several reviews have examined the effectiveness of common interventions used to (1) lessen a child's crying and/or (2) lessen parent anxiety over the child's crying (Joanna Briggs Institute, 2004; Lucassen et al., 1998, 2001). Interventions for colic are often divided into three categories: (1) pharmaceutical interventions, or giving medicine to the infant; (2) dietary interventions, or altering the diet of the child or breast-feeding mother to reduce the existence of certain allergens, and (3) behavioral interventions, or the changing of parent behavior in reaction to the infant's crying (Joanna Briggs Institute, 2004). The Joanna Briggs Institute has evaluated interventions falling under all three of these categories to determine if they could be categorized as being possibly useful, having no effect, or having possibly harmful effects (Joanna Briggs Institute, 2004). "Possibly Useful" interventions have been found to be at least moderately effective across several studies. "No Effect" refers to interventions where either no effect was found or the evidence is very mixed. Finally, the "Possibly Harmful" interventions have evidence of harmful effects or potential harmful effects, as well as limited support for their effectiveness in lessening crying.

According to the Joanna Briggs Institute (2004), there are no pharmaceutical interventions that are potentially useful. In contrast, some medications (Simethicone) have been shown to have no effect, while others may actually be harmful (Anticholinergic drugs, Methylscopolamine). With regard to dietary interventions, several have been shown to be possibly useful (low allergen diet for breast-feeding mother, low allergen formula milk, soy substitute formula milk, and sucrose solution for short term of relief); several other interventions have been shown to have no effect (elimination of cow's milk from breast-feeding mother's diet, lactase supplement/low lactose milk, fiber-enriched formula). Behavioral interventions that have been shown to be possibly useful are reduced stimulation and improved parental responsiveness, while increased carrying, car ride simulators, and focused parent counseling have been shown to have no effect. Early childhood professionals should recommend that families consult with their pediatrician first to address colic; however, knowledge of effective and potentially ineffective or even harmful interventions can help early childhood professionals be prepared to work with families of children with colic.

Colic/Excessive Crying Vignette

Annie has been listening to her 6-week-old daughter Leah cry for over 2 hours. Annie feels upset and frustrated because she has changed Leah's diaper, made sure she did not have gas, and tried to feed her. Realizing her nerves are shot and she needs a break, Annie lays Leah down in her crib, turns on her video baby monitor (with the sound off), and closes the door to Leah's room. Annie decides to take a few minutes for herself and walks outside and sits on her patio drinking hot tea. After 15–20 minutes, Annie is feeling better and returns inside to check on Leah. Although Leah is still crying, Annie reminds herself that this is just a phase that many children go through and it will hopefully be decreasing over the next few weeks.

In addition to these suggestions, another resource is the program *The Period of Purple Crying* (http://www.purplecrying.info/). The website and program was created by the National Center on Shaken Baby Syndrome (NCSBS) and has suggestions for parents to help them cope with the stress of having a child who has colic. The website suggests that colic is typical, although the intensity may vary for each infant, and provides strategies parents can use to both meet their baby's needs and reduce their own stress. The program recommends that after checking to make sure that the baby's needs are met (fed, burped, clean diaper, etc.) and the baby is still crying caregivers should trade off care. If only one caregiver is available, after making sure the baby's needs are met, the caregiver should lay the child down in his or her crib (on his or her back) and take a 15 minutes break to calm himself or herself down. After caregivers are feeling calmer, they can return to their normal caregiving activities. This recommendation comes as a way to prevent Shaken Baby Syndrome, where parents resort to shaking their infant out of frustration over his or her crying.

Toileting Issues

Prevalence

Toilet training is a major milestone achieved by young children and anticipated by parents. Since the 1950s, the age at which children are expected to be potty trained has increased from 2 to 3 years old (Schum et al., 2002). Based on a survey of the parents of approximately 300 children, Schum and colleagues suggest that most children are ready to be potty trained between 22 and 30 months, and most children are able to stay dry during the day just before their third birthday (Schum et al., 2002). Research has suggested that children who start potty training earlier will be potty trained earlier than their peers; however, the process takes longer to complete when started with younger children versus older children (Blum, Taubman, & Nemeth, 2003).

The age at which children are potty trained can vary across genders. Schum et al. (2002) examined the average age that boys and girls are able to engage in different types of toileting behavior ranging from "staying BM-free at night" to "wipes poop effectively by oneself." The study looked at a series of 26 skills and found that girls on average mastered 25 out of 26 toileting skills before boys. The order in which children learned the skills was very similar across genders. Girls were dry during the day by 32 months, while boys met these criteria at 35 months. The lowest level skill in the study ("staying BM-free during the night") occurred on average for girls at 22.1 months and at 24.7 months for boys. The most complex skill of "wiping poop effectively by themselves" occurred at 48.5 months for girls and at 45.1 for boys.

Guidelines

Toilet training will be more successful if parents wait until their child shows global readiness skills, which include both developmental and physical readiness for being trained. The first signs are developmental readiness, such as the child being able to sit on the toilet, understand words for potty functions, and wanting to be independent (Schum et al., 2002). Physical readiness for toilet training includes bladder control and expressed discomfort with soiled diapers (Schum et al., 2002). Even when a child presents these global readiness skills, there may be times when parents might want to postpone toilet training, for example, during major life transitions, such as the birth of a sibling or a move, or during developmental phases when the child is most resistant.

There are a variety of strategies that can be used to promote successful toilet training, which are recommended by the AAP (1999) and Azrin and Foxx's (1974) *Toilet Training in Less Than One Day*. Some parents may prefer the more casual approach recommended by the AAP, during which parents gradually introduce the potty and allow the child to set his or her own schedule. Praise and positive attention make going to the toilet fun; however, one should expect occasional accidents. For others, the Azrin and Fox method is favored, and this involves establishing a regular schedule of sitting on the potty (generally at hourly intervals and after high probability times, such as meals), along with providing positive attention and specific praise. To prepare children to accomplish this major milestone, parents should eliminate diapers and switch to training pants, take their child into the bathroom with them so the child can see what to do, practice with a doll or older sibling, and read books about toileting. Most experts recommend that boys start by sitting on the toilet, and once they understand the concept of using the toilet and have greater physical coordination, they can practice standing. An incentive which works for many boys is to drop Cheerios or bits of toilet paper into the toilet and encourage them to aim.

Fears, Worries, and Anxiety

Prevalence

Fears are common in young children, although variability may occur in terms of how many fears or how intense the reactions to those fears may be. Needleman (2004) reports that, in a survey of parents with preschool age children, over 80 % indicated that their child had at least one fear, while almost 50 % of parents reported that their child had seven or more fears (Needleman, 2004).

Some of the irrational fears that commonly develop in young children (ages 2–6) are thought to increase as a child develops more of an imagination and then gradually decrease as a child becomes more confident and develops cognitive skills to differentiate reality and fantasy (Spencer, 2000). As children grow and develop, they also become more aware of what may go wrong and then worry about such things. The following fears in Table 1.2 are relatively common in young children (Spencer, 2000).

If a child has a fear that is not included in this list, it may also be normal. Sometimes the cause of a fear may be obvious (i.e., the first time at a day care), but it may also be unclear how the fear developed. With the development of fears, parents should be mindful of stressful events such as a move or being left with a new caregiver, which may intensify an existing fear or establish new fears. If a fear seems to be extremely challenging or enduring, the early childhood professional may want to encourage parents to approach their pediatrician or arrange for other

Table 1.2 Common fears in young children

Fear of being left behind/separation anxiety	Fear of loud noises
Fear of dogs or other large animals	Fear of bath time or parts of it
Fear of monsters/witches/clowns/etc.	Fear of flushing toilets
Fear of the dark	Fear of doctors

outside help (Spencer, 2000). At school entry, approximately one in ten children meet the diagnostic criteria for an internalizing disorder (e.g., anxiety and depression; Carter et al., 2010).

Guidelines

Children will outgrow most fears. However, while the child is expressing the fear, it is important to refrain from discounting or invalidating it. General guidelines for addressing fears include gradual exposure to feared event along with support from a nurturing adult, preparing children in advance for stressful situations, teaching them how to relax, and maintaining routines as much as possible. The eventual goal is to increase the child's confidence and coping skills (Spencer, 2000). For example, rather than counteracting a child's fear with reason, parents can join their child and redirect their child's fear in a playful manner (Needleman, 2004). Monsters in the closet can be warded off by spraying "Monster Spray" (a spray bottle of water) toward the closet. These approaches work because most children believe that their parents can protect them and will take care of them.

For fears of separation from the caregiver, it can be helpful to ease children into these transitions so that their anxiety and tension is reduced (Spencer, 2000). This can be accomplished through practicing short separations (i.e., leaving the child with a family member for a few minutes) and having the new caregiver spend time with the child with the primary caregiver present.

For fears of animals and other intimidating figures, early childhood professionals should never force the child to approach or touch the feared object. Instead, build the child's confidence in the situation by having a parent stay close or hold them when the feared object is near, encouraging any approaches (e.g., "Let's have Susie wave at the doggy" and "Look at the clown! He's juggling."). It can also be helpful to role-play how to interact with the feared object by using stuffed animals. If a child fears a cat, practice with a stuffed animal how the child could interact (e.g., "First, the kitty smells our hand. Then, we pet his back.").

Fears of the dark are best handled through a structured bedtime routine that is both relaxing and comforting. This provides a non-anxiety provoking transition into sleeping. If the routine is consistent and fears still are being expressed, early childhood professionals should recommend that parents offer to check on their child in 5–10 min after laying them down (and then follow-through!) or leave the door cracked open with a hall light on. It is not recommended that children be allowed to have the room light on. If a child needs to feel more in control or fears monsters in the dark, parents can give their child a flashlight which is guaranteed to "banish all monsters."

Fears of loud noises can be addressed by explaining the noise (i.e., where thunder comes from) and by remaining calm when the child is fearful so that he or she knows everything is fine. To allow the child more control over the situation, he or she can be encouraged to cover his or her ears to lessen the noise. If a particular object causes the noise (vacuum, hair dryer, etc.), the child can be gradually exposed to the noise, or the use of that object while the child is in the room can be avoided.

Bath time can generate a number of fears such as being sucked down the drain or not feeling in control in a slippery tub. To ease the transition from bath chair to being in the tub, parents can bathe their child with a sponge next to the tub for a little while and then transition to the tub with an inch or two of water. Fears of the bath can also be lessened by encouraging play at bath time with toys or splashing or having parents bathe with their child.

Fears of flushing the toilet may be due to the noise or due to a fear of being sucked down the drain. Parents can choose to not flush the toilet while the child is in the bathroom or can explain that a person is too big to go down the hole at the bottom of the bowl. If this fear is interfering with toilet training, caregivers may opt to have the child use the toddler training toilet and flush the contents after the child has left the bathroom.

Finally, fears of the doctor often appear while a child is a toddler and can vary in intensity. Spencer (2000) offers several recommendations including: (1) have parents obtain and play with a child's pretend doctor's kit and role-play what happens at the doctor's office, (2) encourage parents to allow their child to sit on their lap while at the doctor's, (3) have parents reinforce that the doctor wants to keep the child healthy, (4) have parents tell their child honestly how certain procedures will feel (i.e., "The shot will feel like a pinch and then be all done."), and (5) follow the visit with an enjoyable activity.

Fears Vignette

Samantha is 2½ years old and is going on her first visit to Disney World. She loves all the characters on the Mickey Mouse Club, but her favorite is Goofy. Her parents, Ryan and Sarah, make sure that as soon as they get in the Magic Kingdom, they find out where Goofy will be so Samantha can go see him, get his autograph, and take a picture with him.

Later that day, Samantha and her parents wait 45 min in line for her to see Goofy. Once at the front of the line, Samantha stiffens and tries to get away from Goofy. She is clearly frightened by the six-foot-tall figure before her. Instead of forcing Samantha to stand next to Goofy, Ryan and Sarah take turns getting a picture with Goofy and encourage Samantha to join them. She is still scared and will not approach or look at Goofy. Then, Samantha is encouraged to wave at Goofy and watch as he signs her autograph book. Sarah and Ryan praise Samantha for being so brave and watching Goofy, making sure she feels positive about this interaction.

Sexual Behaviors

Prevalence

Some forms of sexual behavior in young children are common; before children are 13, more than half will have engaged in some type of sexual behavior (Kellogg, 2009). Early childhood professionals must have a clear understanding of what is normal sexual behavior versus what is considered abusive and problematic (National Center on Sexual Behavior of Youth [NCSBY], 2004).

By age 2, children are able to distinguish between boys and girls (Kellogg, 2009). They are naturally interested in body parts, so this is a good time to teach them the names for their genitals. Between the ages of 2 and 5, normal sexual behaviors include touching their genitals in public or private, masturbating, trying to look to see others nude, and showing their genitals to others (Kellogg, 2009). It is less common for children to try to stick their tongue in someone's mouth while kissing, attempt to touch other's genitals, and rub their body against someone else, as these behaviors occur in approximately 8 % of the population (Friedrich, Fisher, Broughton, Houston, & Shafran, 1998). Sexual behaviors in young children tend to increase up through 5 years of age and then gradually decrease, as children become more concerned with privacy (Friedrich et al., 1998).

Some suggest that sexual behaviors are becoming more common in young children as a result of media exposure and cultural changes; however, it is not clear if this increase reflects a change in frequency of sexual behavior or if there is increased awareness of sexual behavior in young children. The NCSBY suggests that sexual behavior is problematic if it includes the following characteristics:

- If it occurs very frequently
- If it interferes with a child's development
- If it includes "coercion, intimidation, or force"
- If there is emotional distress
- If there are big differences in the developmental abilities between the children that are involved
- If after intervention, it occurs frequently in secrecy

Children who experience significant sexual behavior problems (SBPs) are defined as "children 12 years and under who demonstrate developmentally inappropriate or aggressive sexual behavior" (NCSBY, 2004).

If abuse of a child is suspected, early childhood professionals should follow their state law regarding reporting these incidents. In order to make a report it is highly recommended to have the following information on hand (Table 1.3).

Other helpful information includes directions to the victim's location and potential risks to the investigators who will visit the location.

In cases where an early childhood professional may not be sure whether to report or not, it is best to call the state abuse hotline and report the information. The operators receiving the call will assist in the final determination of whether further investigation is necessary.

Table 1.3 Important information to file an abuse report

- A description of the abuse incident, including who was involved, what occurred, when and where it occurred, why it happened, the extent of any injuries, and any other pertinent information
- Names of child and adults involved, along with gender and race/ethnicity information
- Birth date or approximate age of all persons involved
- Addresses for all persons, including current location
- Relationship of the alleged perpetrator to the victim

Guidelines

The NCSBY (2004) suggests that parents do not overreact to sexual behavior in their young children. The attention could inadvertently reinforce the sexual behaviors. The NCSBY also reports that sexual behavior is not a sign that a child has been sexually abused, and some degree of sexual behavior is normal. The NCSBY also suggests that children:

- Should be given the rules regarding sexual behavior (e.g., only masturbate in the privacy of their own room)
- Are taught that sexual behaviors are restricted in some settings
- Are closely supervised
- Are praised for appropriate behavior

Aggression

Prevalence

Aggression is a common problem in young children, and some degree of aggression is typical. Many parents and professionals who work with young children have witnessed aggressive behavior to obtain a desired item (usually a toy that is currently in the hands of a sibling) or to communicate their wants and needs (the sibling then letting the child know that they are not ready to give that particular toy up). Loeber and Stouthamer-Loeber (1998) define aggression as "those acts that inflict bodily or mental harm on others" (p. 242). They also differentiate aggression from violence in that aggressive behaviors do not cause serious harm. In general, aggressive behavior tends to be common in young children and decrease over time. By the time children enter elementary school, externalizing behavior problems, such as aggression, are observed in about 15 % of children (Carter et al., 2010).

The parent–child interaction is one factor that contributes to aggressive behavior in young children. According to Patterson, DeBaryshe, and Ramsey (1989), poor parental discipline, including ignoring appropriate behaviors and allowing aggressive behaviors to escalate, sets the stage for the development of aggressive behaviors. Parental risk factors also contributing to aggressive child behavior include maternal depression, stressful life events, marital conflict, and exposure to violence (Webster-Stratton & Hammond, 1988).

Aggressive behavior is most detrimental to development when it is persistent and stable over time and when it occurs in multiple settings. Miller et al. (1997) report that young children who exhibit aggression at both home and school are more likely to have continued behavioral concerns down the road, compared to those children who are only aggressive at home. Boys are more likely to show aggression than girls. Girls appear to be better at self-regulating their emotions and verbally expressing their feelings. However, at later ages, girls may exhibit other forms of aggression such as shunning and gossiping (Weinberg & Tronick, 1997).

Guidelines

Strategies to decrease challenging behavior, including aggression, are discussed throughout this text. A common component of many parent training programs aimed at reducing aggressive behavior is to increase positive attention for desired behavior and redirect undesired behavior. The idea of "catching your child being good" helps to improve the parent–child relationship and reinforces pro-social behavior rather than aggression. Redirection of negative behaviors helps children learn what is acceptable and what is not, and avoids the negative reinforcement trap, whereby aversive behavior is mistakenly reinforced. Time out is a behavior strategy that when used properly will reduce aggressive behavior and will be discussed in Chap. 6 in more depth. In a nutshell, time out requires a brief removal from the activity in which the child has been aggressive. Time out works because attention is such a powerful motivator for most children. However, one must be mindful of the need to teach children what you want them to do, instead of just punishing them for problematic behaviors.

Numerous studies have shown that spanking has negligible influence on misbehavior. However, it is still used frequently with 26 % of American mothers reporting that they spank their children two or more times per month (Taylor, Manganello, Lee, & Rice, 2010). This is of concern given that spanking appears to increase aggression in children. A study published by Taylor et al. (2010) substantiated that children who were spanked twice or more per month at age 3 were significantly more aggressive by age 5. Spanking teaches a child that the bigger person can control the smaller person by force, and instills fear rather than helping them learn pro-social skills. The AAP does not recommend spanking in any circumstances.

Aggression Vignette

Two and a half-year-old Marcus is happily playing with a ball until he notices his younger brother, Patrick, playing with a toy truck. Quickly, Marcus turns to Patrick, draws back his hand, whacks him on the nose, and immediately grabs the truck. Marcus' display of aggression results in Patrick's wailing cries and Marcus receiving a scolding from his caregivers. This negative attention may inadvertently reinforce aggressive behavior, which may also be reinforced by Marcus obtaining the truck.

Rather than addressing the behavior by scolding, it is recommended that Marcus' caretakers take a different approach. To change his behavior, Marcus' caretakers need to work on "catching him being good" or providing Marcus with positive attention for desired behaviors, redirecting Marcus and providing him opportunities to engage in appropriate behavior, and modeling pro-social behavior, such as sharing and turn-taking.

Social Skills

Prevalence

Social skills refer to the competencies that children need to develop in order to successfully navigate home, school, and community settings (Brown, Odom, & Conroy, 2001). Social skills include behaviors such as sharing, taking turns, using words to express feelings, greeting others, and participating in a group. The most important social skills for preschool age children to master before entering school are listening to others, following classroom rules, compliance with directions, asking for help, cooperating with other children, and controlling their temper (Elliott, Roach, & Beddow, 2008).

Social problems have been found in approximately 14–17 % of young children (Hair & Graziano, 2003; Konold & Pianta, 2005). Children with autism spectrum disorders (ASD) and attention-deficit/hyperactivity disorder (ADHD) are at higher risk for significant social difficulties as they get older. Social difficulties can involve both a lack of skills (e.g., not knowing how to initiate a conversation) and an unwillingness to use skills (e.g., issues related to compliance). As more social demands are placed on children, it is more likely that social difficulties will become more obvious.

Guidelines

The development of social skills in young children is influenced by a number of factors, most importantly, the opportunity to learn and practice social skills. There are several curricula available to teach and reinforce social skills in young children (some evidence-based programs are discussed in Chap. 5). Most follow a similar sequence involving showing the child what to do, helping the child imitate the skills, and providing opportunities to practice in a variety of settings (Elliott et al., 2008). Increasing opportunities for the child to practice these skills during his or her typical daily activities leads to a more natural performance and ensures that the skills become a part of the child's repertoire. In addition, praising and reinforcing these skills when the child uses them will result in these behaviors occurring more frequently.

Social Skills Vignette

Four-year-old Donavan is happily swinging on the swing-set at the park until his caregiver stops pushing him and tells him that it is time to leave. Because Donavan wants to stay he begins to whine. When his caregiver insists that it is time to leave, Donavan's whines quickly turn into screaming and crying. When his caregiver takes his hand to guide him toward the car, he flails his arms around and then runs to the swing-set and wraps his arms and legs around the swing-set pole, continuing to scream and draw attention to himself and his caregiver. In an attempt to stop Donavan's inappropriate behavior, his caregiver lets him swing on the swings until he is ready to leave. Donovan's antisocial behavior may have been reinforced by allowing him to continue to play on the swings, and he may soon learn that by whining, crying, and using physical strength he will not have to comply with adult directives.

Rather than addressing the behavior by giving in to Donavan's demands, it is recommended that Donavan's caregiver take a different approach. Instead of telling him when it is time to leave, Donavan's caregivers should give him warnings when ending a preferred activity, explicitly show him what they want him to do when it is time to end the activity, provide specific positive feedback and praise for following directions, and increase Donavan's opportunities to practice appropriate behavior when transitioning and following directions in a variety of settings.

Cultural Competence

It is important for the early intervention professional to not only be aware of these general guidelines for development but also be prepared to apply these knowledge and skills to children and families from a wide variety of backgrounds and experiences. Recent data suggest that the United States is increasingly culturally and linguistically diverse. For example, 20 % of children in the United States are Latino, approximately 17 % of children in the United States live in poverty, and about 20 %

of school-age children speak a language other than English at home. Cultural competence can help early intervention professionals more effectively meet the needs of the children and families they work with and improve the quality of services and outcomes.

Culture has been defined as "An integrated pattern of human behavior that includes thoughts, communications, languages, practices, beliefs, values, customs, courtesies, rituals, manners of interacting and roles, relationships and expected behaviors of a racial, ethnic, religious or social group; and the ability to transmit the above to succeeding generations" (National Center for Cultural Competence of Georgetown University, http://gucchd.georgetown.edu/nccc/). As this definition implies, culture is multidimensional and cultural competence requires a significant level of knowledge and understanding. The knowledge and skills to work effectively with children and families from all kinds of backgrounds is essential to being an effective early childhood professional.

The development of cultural competence is something that takes time, effort, and experience, and will be an ongoing process for the early intervention professional. A comprehensive discussion of this topic is beyond the scope of this text; however, we will present a model of cultural competence that involves awareness, reflection, and knowledge (National Association for the Education of Young Children [NAEYC], 1996; Wright Carroll, 2009). This model provides guidance in working effectively with culturally and linguistically diverse children and families.

Step 1: Awareness

Early intervention professionals must be aware of their own cultural perspectives and beliefs. Wright Carroll (2009) suggests that this step includes awareness of personal values and beliefs, awareness of other's beliefs, awareness that individuals have multiple cultural identities, and awareness of systemic cultural issues such as privilege and exclusion. One of the keys to awareness is to consider the multiple identities that we have, as well as to recognize that other's perspectives will be framed by a variety of cultural experiences.

Step 2: Reflection

As a second step, the professionals are encouraged to reflect upon how their own background and identity impact how they interact with young children and their families. Early intervention professionals should recognize when their knowledge and actions are not consistent with best practices or do not demonstrate cultural competency and take steps to increase their awareness and knowledge when this occurs.

Step 3: Knowledge

Another component of cultural competency is having an understanding of the cultural and linguistic backgrounds of those children and families that a professional works with. This knowledge can be helpful in how to approach children and families, as well as how to interpret other's actions. However, at this step it is also critical to not overgeneralize knowledge of group characteristics to individual children and families. Each child's and family's background will be the result of their unique experiences, just as an early childhood professional's cultural and linguistic identity is multidimensional.

This framework provides the early childhood professional with guidelines to follow when working with children and families. We have provided some additional resources below.

National Center for Cultural Competence
http://www11.georgetown.edu/research/gucchd/nccc/
This site has a lot of educational materials, as well as self assessments of cultural competence

U.S. Department of Health and Human Services
National Standards on Culturally and Linguistically Appropriate Services (CLAS)
http://minorityhealth.hhs.gov/templates/browse.aspx?lvl=2&lvlID=15

American Academy of Pediatrics
Policy Statement: Ensuring Culturally Effective Pediatric Care—Implications for Education and Health
http://aappolicy.aappublications.org/cgi/content/full/pediatrics;114/6/1677

Conclusions

Challenging behavior is quite common in young children, especially emerging around the second year of life. Parents are often concerned about whether or not their child's behavior is normal, how to handle behavior problems, and where to seek help. In fact, one study found that 70 % of mothers were more worried about their parenting than about their own health (Hickson, Altemeler, & O'Connor, 1983). Furthermore, the availability of information and misinformation, via the internet and other media sources, can lead to further confusion at a time when parents need to decide upon a course of action. A well-informed early childhood professional can assist parents and other caregivers during this very crucial time, when toddlers are naturally testing the limits and forming their personalities, by providing guidance in positive methods that have a high likelihood of working, such as implementing consistent routines, providing specific praise and attention for desired behavior, preventing or redirecting problem behavior, and using time out infrequently and only when the child is able to understand. The relationship and partnership established between the professional and the parent will provide the foundation to promote parenting skills that will strengthen the family and ultimately lead to optimal child outcomes.

Assess Your Knowledge

Use the questions below to assess your knowledge of the information presented in this chapter. Answers appear after the last question.

1. Why is it important to know if a child is experiencing sleep difficulties?

   a. Inadequate sleep has been linked to health and behavior problems, including academic, social, and emotional difficulties.
   b. Inadequate sleep is common in young children.
   c. Many children do not receive adequate treatment for their sleep problems.
   d. All of the above.

2. A parent of a 20-month-old girl tells you that they would like to potty train their daughter. Compared to the typical age that children are potty trained, you might tell them that:

   a. They should begin potty training their daughter immediately.
   b. They should consider whether their daughter has demonstrated global readiness skills.
   c. Children cannot be potty trained until 3 years of age.
   d. Children will tell you when they are ready to be potty trained.

3. How many hours of sleep are recommended for an 18-month-old child within a 24-hour period?

   a. 14–16 h
   b. 9–12 h
   c. 8–10 h
   d. 12–14 h

4. Giving in to an aggressive child's demands is likely to:

   a. Discourage the child from engaging in aggressive behavior in the future.
   b. Encourage the child to engage in aggressive behavior in the future.
   c. Not change the aggressive behavior.
   d. Make the child mad.

5. Which one of the following behaviors is a common sexual behavior in children ages 2–5?

   a. Masturbating
   b. French kissing
   c. Touching other's genitals
   d. Forcing another child to touch their genitals

6. Beginning at age 2, it is recommended by the USDA that children eat the following types of foods:

   a. Six servings of Grain food group, 3 from the Vegetable food group, 2 from the Fruit group, 2 from the Milk group, and 2 from the Meat and Beans Group.
   b. Six servings of Grain food group, 0 from the Vegetable food group, 1 from the Fruit group, 2 from the Milk group, and 2 from the Meat and Beans Group.
   c. Ten servings of Grain food group, 10 from the Vegetable food group, 10 from the Fruit group, 10 from the Milk group, and 10 from the Meat and Beans Group.
   d. Four servings of Grain food group, 3 from the Vegetable food group, 2 from the Fruit group, 3 from the Milk group, and 5 from the Meat and Beans Group.

7. Which of the following choices is NOT a recommendation for parents regarding how to deal with sexual behaviors in their young child?

   a. Children should be given the rules regarding sexual behavior (e.g., only masturbate in the privacy of their own room).
   b. Children should be taught that sexual behaviors is restricted in some settings.
   c. Parents should immediately draw attention to their children when they engage in sexual behavior.
   d. Children should be closely supervised.

8. Which of the following is NOT a guideline for dealing with eating issues in your child?

   a. Force-feed your child when they don't eat.
   b. Make mealtime structured with regard to the timing and seating requirements.
   c. Always serve milk with meals.
   d. Avoid making special meals for children who are picky.

9. Social skills are best taught to children

   a. In the therapist's office, where you have more control over the environment.
   b. When a child is in the middle of a tantrum.
   c. In everyday routines.
   d. Who know what to do, but choose not to do it.

10. Spanking as a disciplinary consequence is

    a. Very effective with young children in the long term.
    b. May temporarily stop the behavior.
    c. Useful to get a child's attention.
    d. Is the recommended consequence for aggressive behavior.

Assess Your Knowledge Answers
1) d   2) b   3) d   4) b   5) a   6) a   7) c   8) a   9) c   10) b

Chapter 2
Early Childhood Development Theories

Abstract Developmental theories are useful towards understanding how children learn and grow, and by what means their trajectories can be supported. Most theorists agree that both biology and experience are key factors that shape developmental outcomes. Risk and protective factors are said to contribute to development and often can be modified through intervention efforts. The prevention model emphasizes a foundation of supports and services aimed to foster healthy development.

Keywords Secure base behavior • Emotional regulation • Egocentric • Accommodation • Assimilation • Equilibrium • Zone of proximal development • Positive reinforcement • Negative reinforcement • Punishment • Parenting styles • Modeling • Ecological theory • Risk and protective factors • Prevention model

Theories of development provide a framework for thinking about human growth, development, and learning. If you have ever wondered about what motivates human thought and behavior or how personalities form, understanding these theories can provide useful insight into both the individual and societal influences on early development. The next section will briefly review the major developmental theories that help to explain how development unfolds, sources of vulnerability and protection that influence child development, and how the course of development may be altered by prevention and intervention efforts. Understanding factors which may support or compromise development and integrating this knowledge into one's work with children and their families are key to supporting healthy developmental outcomes and creating trusting partnerships with caregivers. This chapter will begin with attachment theory, and will provide an overview of the basic concepts proposed by the major developmental theories, which can be utilized by the early childhood professional in screening, assessing, and intervening with young children and their families.

K.H. Armstrong et al., *Evidence-Based Interventions for Children with Challenging Behavior*, DOI 10.1007/978-1-4614-7807-2_2, © Springer Science+Business Media New York 2014

Attachment Theory

Attachment theory is rooted in the joint work of John Bowlby and Mary Ainsworth, whose research first documented the importance of the relationship that developed between the mother and her child. Additionally, this research helped to document the detrimental impact upon children's development resulting from parental separation, deprivation, or bereavement (Ainsworth & Bowlby, 1991). Attachment is thought to be developed in phases, beginning before birth, when mothers first develop emotional feelings for their unborn babies. Attachment is believed to be a lifelong process, involving both intimacy and independence.

Newborn babies have been described as "wired for feelings and ready to learn" (National Research Council and Institute of Medicine [NRCIM], 2000, p. 4), and advances in research about early brain development support the importance of nurturing during the earliest years of life (NRCIM, 2000). In the first 2 months after birth, the baby and his or her caregivers must adjust and adapt to the changes brought on by the baby's first few weeks at home. During the early attachment phase, the baby learns to signal caregivers, who in return, respond to the baby's needs for food and comfort. *Emotional regulation* is a process whereby the infant learns to manage stressful situations through interactions with his or her caregivers, which eventually helps the infant to self-sooth. The quality of early caregiving is thought to either assist or impede the infant's ability to regulate inner emotional states; when the caregiver responds consistently to the baby's signals, the baby begins to develop a sense of competence and enjoys social interactions.

By 2–7 months of life, the baby's feeding and sleeping cycles are becoming more regulated and predictable. Babies are more interactive, easier to care for, and will smile at their caregivers. By 6 months of age, babies show differentiated emotions of joy, surprise, sadness, disgust, and anger, respond to the emotional expressions of others, and enjoy turn-taking vocalizing. Around 7–9 months of age, the preference for familiar caregivers and protests around separation from them emerges and is referred to as *separation anxiety*. When babies become "attached," they become increasingly wary and anxious around strangers, and it becomes even more important for the caregiver to offer comfort, nurturance, and protection. Babies become attached to caregivers with whom they have had significant amounts of interaction. Caregivers are described as being hierarchically arranged in terms of preference, so that the baby has a most preferred caregiver, a next most preferred caregiver, etc.; however, there is thought to be a limit to the attachment capacity. Serious attachment disturbances become evident in settings where babies have to depend upon large numbers of caregivers, such as in institutions, or when there are frequent disruptions of caregivers, such as in foster care placements (Smyke, Dumitrescu, & Zeanah, 2002).

The concept of *secure base behavior*, which emerges during toddlerhood (12–20 months), describes the willingness of the child to venture out from the caregiver to safely explore the world (Ainsworth & Bowlby, 1991). Secure base behavior develops along with the toddler's ability to walk and explore and the toddler's new sense of will. A toddler's ability to say "no" demonstrates that he or she has developed a solid sense of self as separate from the caregiver. The caregiver must learn to guide the child's behavior by setting limits firmly and lovingly to keep the toddler safe and secure. At the same time, the caregiver must reinforce and build the child's self-confidence through positive reinforcement.

Between 20 and 24 months, the toddler's attachment continues to evolve to others outside of the immediate family through exposure to new experiences in community settings such as daycares. Communication and play skills become more developed and complex. Securely attached children are described as more autonomous, socially confident, flexible in problem solving, and affectionate. By age 3, such children are described as empathetic, have better social skills, and have become good communicators. In summary, attachment theory posits that early human relationships and experiences lay the foundation for later development and learning.

Attachment Theory Vignette

Two-year-old Maya has recently begun squirming and saying "no" when mother tries to secure her in her car seat. Maya has begun to develop a sense of self and autonomy, separate from her caregivers. Her caregivers must consistently set limits and follow through with Maya, to keep her safe and secure while riding in the car. They can increase her willingness to comply by providing specific praise along with a special toy to hold whenever she gets into her car seat without resistance.

Cognitive Theory

Certainly, anyone trained to work with young children has come across the work of Jean Piaget. Piaget is best known for his theory of cognitive development in children, which proposed that children's cognitive skills progress through a series of stages in which new information from experiences is taken in and understood. Stages in early childhood development include the sensori-motor (ages birth to 24 months) and preoperational (ages 2–6 years) periods. In the sensori-motor period, children learn to coordinate and repeat actions which are pleasurable. They also begin to understand that symbols (words) can represent objects or events and to comprehend the concept of *object permanence*, meaning that objects continue to exist, even when not visible. In the preoperational period, language becomes the hallmark of development. Children begin to engage in pretend play and will take on roles such as Mommy or Daddy. However, they are still *egocentric*, or unable to take the view of another person.

Piaget believed that from birth, children are driven to explore and master their own environment, take pleasure in mastery, and develop self-confidence through doing. Children learn by taking in new information (*assimilation*), which adds to and changes (*accommodation*) their prior understanding and knowledge (*schemas*). For example, if a child's experience has been with small dogs, she might believe that all dogs are furry, have four legs, bark, and are small. When she encounters a big dog, she must take in the new information and modify her existing schema so that it makes sense. Piaget explained that children must strike a balance between assimilation and accommodation (*equilibrium*), and in doing so, are able to move from one stage of thought to the next stage. Thus, children in the sensori-motor and preoperational stages of development must have experiences and opportunities to learn new information and concepts. Caregivers can facilitate children's learning by providing them ample opportunities to explore and by monitoring them to keep them safe.

The insights offered by psychologist Lev Vygotsky are also important to consider in working with young children. Vygotsky coined the term *zone of proximal development*, which refers to the ideal level of adult/older child support or assistance that a child needs to learn a new skill. *Scaffolding* refers to the adjustment that one must make with supports, in order to enhance the child's independence and confidence in learning new skills. Like Piaget, Vygotsky emphasized the importance of play in learning new language and cognitive skills, and along with attachment theorists believed that play enhanced social development. Play becomes the vehicle through which children learn and internalize social rules, which develops self-regulation, and relationships with others (Vygotsky, 1978).

Applied Behavior Analysis

Applied behavior analysis (ABA) has been referred to as "the science devoted to the understanding and improvement of human behavior" (Cooper, Heron, & Heward, 2007, p. 3). Behavior is understood by observing the relationship of behavior to the environment, which incorporates rules governing learning and maintenance of behaviors. ABA always involves careful measurement of behavior and its consequences, and utilizes behavioral technology to strengthen desired behaviors and to weaken undesirable behaviors. Other terms for ABA include learning theory (most often used in educational settings), behaviorism (associated mostly with Skinner and early pioneers in this field), and behavior modification. Positive Behavior Support (PBS) emerged from ABA and emphasizes the prevention of inappropriate behavior, understanding the function of behavior, redirection of problem behaviors, and teaching replacement skills. ABA has been used successfully with individuals of all ages and abilities, and is implemented across settings such as home, school, or other community settings.

Behavior, by definition, must be observable and measurable, and includes both reflexive and operant behaviors. Reflexive behaviors are those which automatically occur. Reflexive behaviors can also become linked to a neutral stimulus. For example, a dog will automatically salivate to food; however, if one rings a bell right before feeding a dog, the dog will eventually salivate to the sound of the bell, even without the food being presented. In fact, the dog may even salivate when a doorbell rings, a timer goes off, or to anything similar to the bell, and this is called *generalization*. However, if one continues to ring the bell over a period of time and does not present food, the dog will no longer salivate, which is called *extinction*. This technology is used to help people overcome fears or anxiety responses, by gradually exposing them to anxiety-evoking events, while teaching them to relax.

Operant behaviors refer to behaviors as they are maintained by consequences, or the outcomes of the behavior. If the behavior is increased, the consequence is referred to as reinforcement. Positive reinforcement includes consequences such as food, attention, or activities that increase the probability that the behavior will reoccur. An example of positive reinforcement is praise for desired behavior. Negative reinforcement refers to consequences which are avoided through the behavior. For example, a driver may slow down when he notices a police car ahead of him. This behavior results in avoiding a ticket, which increases the likelihood of slowing down in the presence of a police car in the future. Punishment is a consequence that may temporarily stop a behavior from occurring; for example, if the driver is ticketed for speeding, he may slow down for a while. Extinction refers to a process of withholding reinforcement that has maintained behavior, which will lead to a decline of the behavior. Ignoring unwanted behavior will gradually extinguish that behavior if practiced consistently.

Shaping refers to a process of teaching new skills through the process of reinforcement. By breaking down the desired behavior into simple skills, and reinforcing each skill, the desired goal will eventually be reached. If there is also undesired behavior, one may consider combining reinforcement and extinction; for example, ignoring undesirable behavior, while reinforcing desired behavior, will eventually result in increases of desired behavior.

Schools have utilized principles of ABA not only to address challenging behaviors once they have occurred but also to prevent these behaviors from occurring in the first place. School-wide PBS combines ABA technology within a prevention framework, such that all students benefit from school-wide supports such as social skills training, while those students with more intensive needs receive the attention that they require to be successful (Sugai & Horner, 2005). This model has been successfully implemented in early childhood through high school settings and emphasizes the following:

- Proactive instructional approaches to teaching and improving social behaviors
- Conceptually sound and empirically validated practices
- Systems change to support effective practices
- Data-based decision making

For young children, and children with disabilities, the following PBS strategies are endorsed (Fox, Carta, Strain, Dunlap, & Hemmeter, 2010):

- Functional Behavioral Assessment and assessment-based interventions
- Functional communication training
- Self-management/monitoring
- Choice making

Social learning theory emerged from learning theory and helps to explain how new behavior may be learned simply by watching others (Bandura, 1977). Social learning theory is also known as modeling or vicarious learning. Through the controversial Bobo Doll experiments, Bandura proved that young children exposed to televised aggression became more aggressive, even though their behaviors had not been reinforced through consequences. Social learning is thought to be influenced by internal processes involving attention, memory, and motivation, which might not be as readily observable as behavior and its consequences. Young children are especially attuned to learning through modeling or watching others, especially if they identify with the model, or see that the model is reinforced for its actions. Thus, aggressive and violent actions shown by cartoon characters or other media and seen by children may actually influence children to behave in similar ways, especially if the character is reinforced for its actions.

Social Learning Vignette

Four-year-old Justin watched a wrestling match with his parents and older siblings. His family cheered, clapped, and high-fived whenever their favorite wrestler punched or kicked his opponent. A few days later, Justin's teacher reported to his parents that he was punching and kicking his friends at school. They could not understand why Justin began displaying these aggressive behaviors, because they did not allow punching or kicking at home.

Social learning theory helps us to understand how Justin learned these aggressive behaviors. He witnessed aggressive behavior at the wrestling match, identified with the wrestler, and saw his family and others reinforce the wrestler for his aggressive actions by clapping and cheering.

Parenting Styles

Parenting styles is a concept first described by Diana Baumrind (1966) and later expanded by Maccoby and Martin (1983). It refers to the degree to which parents respond to their child's needs, disciplinary strategies they use, parental expectations for maturity and control, and the effects that this has on their child's development. There are four styles of parenting:

1. *Authoritarian*, or "too hard," parenting style is described as highly demanding but not responsive parenting. Children are expected to follow strict rules, and not following rules will result in punishment. These parents value obedience, tradition, and order, and expect children to obey without questioning. This type of parenting style may lead to children who are obedient and proficient, but less happy and self-confident. In extreme cases, abusive parents may fall in this category.

2. *Permissive*, or "too soft," parenting style is depicted as low demands, but highly responsive. Parents, who are permissive, place few demands on the child, allow the child to regulate his or her own behavior, and remain nurturing and communicative. Parents take on the role more of a friend than a parent. This may lead to children who seem spoiled or self-centered, and they do not perform as well in school.

3. *Authoritative*, or "just right," parenting style is portrayed as moderately demanding and responsive. Authoritative parents set and reinforce limits, but are much more responsive and willing to listen to questions. When children fail to meet expectations, they are more likely to be forgiving instead of punishing, and see discipline as teaching. Children of authoritative parents are thought to be the most happy, capable, and successful.

4. *Uninvolved* parenting style is characterized by few demands, low responsiveness, and little communication. These parents seem to be detached from their child's life and, in extreme cases, may neglect or reject their child. Their children may lack self-control, have lower self-esteem, and are less competent than peers.

Various researchers have supported the authoritative parenting style as being the most beneficial towards raising happy, confident, and capable children (Baumrind, 1991; Guzell & Vernon-Feagans, 2004; Neary & Eyberg, 2002). As such, the authoritative parenting style is the most often included in the evidence-based parenting programs.

Ecological Systems Theory

Ecological systems theory was proposed by Urie Bronfenbrenner (1979) to help explain how children develop within the context of their world. He described five systems that influence development, Microsystem, Mesosystem, Exosystem, Macrosystem, and Chronosystem, and considered that the person's biology also contributed to this system. Thus, both environmental and biological factors are thought to shape development and child outcomes. Bronfenbrenner is one of the founders of the Head Start Program, a federal program intended to improve cognitive and developmental outcomes for children and their families from low income backgrounds through education, health, nutrition, and parent training efforts.

The concept of risk and protective factors emerges out of ecological systems theory. Those features which are thought to contribute to behavioral disorders and poor developmental outcomes are defined as *risk factors*. Risk factors, which are biological in nature, reside within the child and include prenatal exposure to substances, premature birth, temperament, developmental delays, chronic medical conditions, and insecure attachments. Environmental risk factors, or those which are external to the child, include factors such as inconsistent caregiving, poverty, abuse, and neglect.

Protective factors, on the other hand, are thought to improve self-regulation and behavior and, again, may be described as within-child factors and external factors. Within-child protective factors include health and wellness, high cognitive skills, and strong adaptive skills. External protective factors include warm and predictable caregiving relationships, safe experiences and environments, and firm and consistent discipline, as well as community supports, health services, schools, laws, etc.

Prevention Model

Concerns about young children's health and well-being have caused researchers and practitioners to think in terms of prevention. The public health prevention model emphasizes multiple layers of supports and services aimed to decrease risk factors and reduce disorders, in order to promote better outcomes (Kazak, 2006). In the case of young children, the principle of nurturing environments is proposed to prevent multiple problems and improve success (Mercy & Saul, 2009). *Primary prevention* refers to efforts which target all children and families. An example of primary prevention would be the Back-to-Sleep campaign, which is intended to reduce infant deaths due to Sudden Infant Death Syndrome or SIDS. *Secondary prevention/intervention* is more intensive and is targeted towards at-risk populations, with Head Start being a prime example as it supports young children at risk for school failure due to poverty. *Tertiary prevention/intervention* is considered to be the most intensive support within the prevention model, and intended for children and their families who are already experiencing significant difficulties. Federal special education and early intervention are examples of tertiary prevention/intervention, as only the most at-risk are eligible for those services, and the intention is to prevent further damage and improve outcomes.

The prevention framework allows for greater efficiency in how service delivery is organized, delivered, and funded, with the most intensive services reserved for the most at-risk. This framework is called by different names depending upon the system of care in which it operates; among them are *Recognition and Response* (Coleman, Buysse, & Neitzel, 2006), *Teaching Pyramid* (Fox et al., 2010), *Stepped Care* (Bower & Gilbody, 2005), *Nurturing Environments* (Komro, Flay, & Biglan, 2011), and *Response to Intervention* (Van Der Heyden & Snyder, 2006). Each of these models describes supports and services in a three- or four-tiered model which describe the most effective and efficient methods of preventing and treating problems. In the remaining chapters, the prevention model will provide the framework in discussions about how to integrate research, experience, and best practice efforts towards fostering positive outcomes and reducing behavior problems in the young children.

Conclusions

This chapter highlights theories of development that help explain how children learn and grow, by what means their behavior may be modified and improved, and why it is argued that their outcomes are shaped by both biology and experiences.

Understanding factors which may support or compromise development and integrating this knowledge into one's work with children and their families are crucial towards cultivating more supportive environments. The early childhood professional can help parents and other caregivers by teaching them how to spend more enjoyable time with their child, reinforce positive skills, monitor behavior and set limits, and reduce the use of harsh discipline methods. These are the essential parenting skills that help children develop prosocial behavior, self-regulation, and other skills they will need to be successful in school and other settings.

Assess Your Knowledge

Use this vignette to answer questions 1–7.

Maria (age 3) asks Juan (age 24 months) to share a toy, but he loudly protests and throws himself on the floor. The early intervention practitioner intervenes, making this a teaching moment for both children and their parent. For each question (1–7), circle the letter that best describes the theory underlying this approach.

1. The practitioner ignores Juan and praise Maria for using her words.

   a. Attachment theory
   b. Cognitive theory
   c. Behavior (reinforcement) theory
   d. Authoritarian Parenting

2. The practitioner offers Maria another toy and says "I'll share with you. Sharing is fun."

   a. Accommodation
   b. Modeling
   c. Authoritative Parenting
   d. Emotional regulation

3. The practitioner says to Juan "Oh…I can see that you don't want to share right now. It's your special toy."

   a. Cognitive theory
   b. Modeling and imitation
   c. Permissive parenting
   d. Prevention model

4. The practitioner pays no attention to both children and looks at Facebook with parent.

   a. Negative reinforcement
   b. Authoritative parenting
   c. Uninvolved parenting
   d. Permissive parenting

5. The practitioner says to Juan "When you have finished with the toy, please give it to Maria for a little while."

   a. Cognitive theory
   b. Authoritative parenting
   c. Authoritarian parenting
   d. Permissive parenting

6. The practitioner reprimands and sends both children to corner for not sharing.

   a. Behavior (reinforcement) theory
   b. Authoritative parenting
   c. Authoritarian parenting
   d. Uninvolved parenting

7. Perhaps Juan is not mature enough to understand sharing. The practitioner decides to practice an activity, such as tossing a ball back and forth, which requires turn taking and sharing.

   a. Cognitive theory
   b. Authoritarian parenting
   c. Permissive parenting
   d. Ecological model

8. Little Albert is playing with a stuffed bunny when someone pops a gun behind him. Now he cries whenever he sees any kind of a stuffed animal or pet. This is an example of:

   a. Immaturity
   b. Attention seeking behavior
   c. Generalization
   d. Egocentricity

9. You decide to run a 5 km race, but you cannot walk more than a mile without feeling exhausted. You set up a schedule for yourself, beginning with a mile walk and gradually increasing your walking distance until you reach your goal. This is an example of:

   a. Prevention
   b. Shaping
   c. Equilibrium
   d. Modeling

10. Aysha was born at 25 weeks gestation. Her mother is 17 years old and has dropped out of school. We might think of these as:

    a. Uninvolved parenting
    b. Negative reinforcement
    c. Risk factors
    d. Generalization

Assess Your Knowledge Answers
1) c   2) b   3) c   4) c   5) d   6) c   7) a   8) c   9) b   10) c

Chapter 3
The Prevention Model and Problem Solving

Abstract With growing numbers of developmental needs expressed in communities, the way services are delivered to families must change to assist children. A prevention model which provides multiple levels of support from prevention efforts to extensive, individualized interventions can assist practitioners in meeting the needs of children efficiently and effectively. In addition, prevention and intervention efforts are more effective when problems are clearly identified and tied to specific interventions which are evidence-based. The use of a problem-solving process gives practitioners a specific way to think about child concerns and develop and track progress of interventions matched to the child or children's needs.

Keywords Primary prevention • Secondary prevention/intervention • Tertiary prevention/intervention • Problem-solving process • Problem identification • Problem analysis • Intervention implementation • Intervention evaluation • Collaborative problem solving

A need for children's services and support in communities across the United States is prominent. Approximately 1 in 5 children in the United States have a diagnosable behavioral health disorder and current statistics indicate that only 20 % of children with severe behavioral health concerns will receive any kind of assistance (Society for Research in Child Development, 2009; U.S. Public Health Service, 2001). These problems when left unaddressed can negatively affect their functioning and development (Brauner & Stephens, 2006). With such a large need present and a limited number of qualified professionals to meet the need, communities must adopt an efficient model of service delivery. By matching the intensity of a service with the needs of a family, more children can be helped to reach developmental milestones on time. In the next section, a tiered service delivery model, identified as the prevention model, is described. This model focuses on prevention and early intervention to promote positive outcomes.

K.H. Armstrong et al., *Evidence-Based Interventions for Children with Challenging Behavior*, DOI 10.1007/978-1-4614-7807-2_3,
© Springer Science+Business Media New York 2014

Primary Prevention

Primary prevention, also referred to as Universal, efforts consist of enhancing protective factors in families and community settings and are designed to prevent the future development of more negative child and family outcomes. An example of primary prevention is the *Back to Sleep* campaign, which is a public service campaign that is designed to educate all parents and caregivers about the importance of putting babies to sleep on their backs to prevent sudden infant death syndrome (SIDS). Prevention efforts can consist of general support and information provided through handouts or public service announcements. A key idea within primary prevention is to provide educational information to people who care for and/or work with children, so that they will be better informed about how to best promote healthy development. The guidelines presented in Chap. 1 for common behavior problems are examples of primary prevention efforts because all young children will benefit when those guidelines are followed. In the case of older children, school-wide social skills programs are considered to be primary prevention efforts because all children will benefit from social skills instruction. Primary prevention requires relatively little time and cost relative to individual intervention efforts, and is accessible to everyone in the community. Although some children and families will need more intensive interventions as well, the needs of 80–90 % of children and families are expected to be met with these low cost efforts. High quality, primary prevention efforts are also important as they can reserve resources to develop and provide services and supports to children and families in significant need.

Secondary Prevention/Intervention

Secondary prevention, also referred to as Targeted, involves activities slated for children who may develop problem behaviors as a result of certain risk factors, and as such need programs tailored to promote their success. Children growing up in poverty are an example of individuals for whom secondary prevention efforts such as developmentally appropriate preschool experiences can result in positive outcomes such as improved readiness for school. Secondary prevention activities are provided in groups and are often implemented through educational, health care, or social services. Head Start is an example of a federally funded secondary prevention endeavor that promotes school readiness and cognitive gains through the provision of educational, health, nutritional, social, and other services. Children and families are eligible for Head Start based upon income status and/or disability, thus targeting the needs of approximately 5–15 % of children. The Nurse–Family Partnership is another secondary prevention approach, in that it targets low income, first-time mothers and provides them with healthcare and development guidance.

Group parent training programs are yet another example of secondary prevention efforts, as they provide caregivers with information and support to improve parent–child relationships and proactive discipline skills.

Tertiary Prevention/Intervention

Lastly, tertiary prevention, or Clinical/treatment, includes more intensive and individualized supports for children with chronic issues and their families. As healthy development in young children includes both physical and mental health, these services are generally delivered by an interdisciplinary team and often across systems of care. Ideally, tertiary prevention/intervention will only be required by 5 % of families if quality primary and secondary prevention strategies are in place and accessible to families. Tertiary strategies should be aimed to maximize development and improve functioning, and as such, may prevent a problem from becoming worse or a related problem from developing. An example of tertiary prevention/intervention efforts would be Part C of The *Individuals with Disabilities Education Act (IDEA)* a federal law ensuring services to children birth to three with delays and/or disabilities. Over 6.5 million eligible infants, toddlers, children, and youth with disabilities are covered under this legislation (Retrieved December 10, 2012 from http://www2.ed.gov/policy/speced/reg/idea/part-c/index.html). Each child and family eligible for Part C services will receive an Individual Family Support Plan (IFSP) which documents developmental goals, objectives and outcomes, as well as age-appropriate services and supports for the child and family. Another example of tertiary efforts would be individual behavioral health services needed for children with significant disruptive behaviors that resulted in their suspension from daycare or preschool, and are designed to help them thrive in such environments. Children who have experienced trauma or chronic illness are another group who might need extensive evaluation and support from a mental health professional to improve coping strategies.

Matching the Level of Care to the Child and Family's Needs

The prevention model is often depicted as a pyramid, in which one thinks about how to prevent and intervene with developmental problems:

- *Tertiary prevention/intervention*: Smallest number of children/families who require more extensive support and therapeutic services.
- *Secondary prevention/intervention*: Higher risk children and families need increased support and guidance to strengthen their coping skills.
- *Primary prevention*: Most children and families benefit from general information and support.

Problem-Solving Process Embedded in the Prevention Model

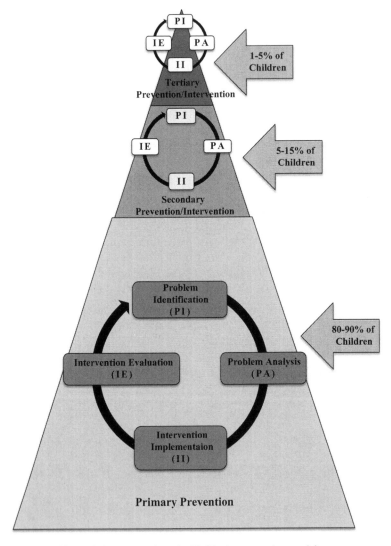

Fig. 3.1 The problem-solving process is embedded in the prevention model

Four-step problem-solving process:

1. **Problem identification**—*Is there a problem? What is it?*

    (a) Sub-step 1: Define the problem in specific behavioral terms

    - What does the behavior look like?
    - When did the behavior occur?
    - What was the child doing?
    - Who else was present and what were they doing?

    (b) Sub-step 2: Define the desired behavior in specific behavioral terms

    - What is the desired or replacement behavior?
    - What skills are needed to reach desired behavior goal?

    (c) Sub-step 3: Determine where the child's behavior falls in comparison to age expectations (this is also called Gap Analysis)

    - How does the child's present behavior compare to expectations for her age?
    - These expectations are also referred to as benchmarks or milestones.

    There are several methods one might use to help identify the problem, including structured interviews, screening tools, standardized rating scales, observations, and/or other assessments.

2. **Problem analysis**—*Why is the problem happening?*

    (a) The purpose of this step is to develop multiple hypotheses to explain why the child is not exhibiting the desired behavior.
    (b) Hypothesis Format: (Child) does (problem behavior) because…
    (c) It is important to think about the environment in which the child lives, family relationships and support systems, and health factors that may be contributing to the problem.

3. **Intervention implementation**—*What will be done about the problem? Who will do it? How often and for how long will they do it? How will we know if the intervention is working?*

    (a) Using the information gathered through problem analysis, interventions are selected/developed and implemented.
    (b) The interventions should be closely aligned with the hypothesis for why the problem is occurring. For example, two children who exhibit tantrum behavior may have different reasons for doing this (Anthony: to get attention, Sarah: because she does not have the language to express her needs), and the interventions that would be most likely to be successful should match to the specific hypotheses. An intervention to address Anthony's tantrums may focus on strategies to seek attention appropriately and his parents may need to ignore tantrums. For Sarah, an intervention to increase her ability to

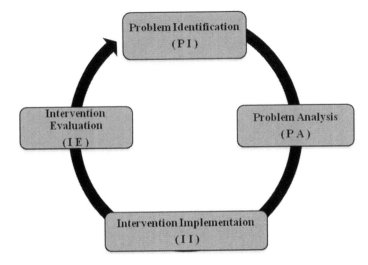

Fig. 3.2 The four-step problem-solving process

express her needs (e.g., teaching her words or sign) would be more likely to be effective.

(c) The following information must be specified in the plan:

- *Who* will do *what*?
- *When* it will be done?
- *How* long will it be tried?

(d) Also included in this step is determining the data collection method, which will be needed to monitor the response to the intervention.

- *How* will we know if the intervention is working?
- *When* will the intervention be evaluated?

4. **Intervention evaluation**—*Is the intervention working?*

(a) This step involves revisiting the problem originally identified and examining data to determine if the intervention is working.

(b) A determination is made (based on the data) whether the intervention needs to continue, be modified, or be discontinued.

(c) If the problem persists, the problem-solving process must be repeated in order to redesign a more effective intervention. New information is gleaned throughout the problem-solving process which can be used to better understand the problem and informing more effective future iterations of the intervention.

The problem-solving process appears in Fig. 3.2. and is applied in a case study in Table 3.1.

Table 3.1 Case study using the problem-solving process

Background Information: Ethan is 2 years old and has met most of his developmental milestones. Ethan's mother is concerned because he is not talking as much as his older sister did at 2 years old	
Problem identification	Through questioning it is determined that Ethan is delayed with respect to communication milestones. He has a vocabulary of about 10–15 words and does not utter any phrases. Communication milestones at age 2 include a vocabulary of at least 200 words, speaking in 2–4 word phrases, speech that is 50 % intelligible, naming six body parts, and following simple directions. Ethan can follow simple directions, turns to his name, and points to his body parts. Thus, we have determined that Ethan is showing a delay of about 6 months in expressive communication
Problem analysis	Further questioning reveals that Ethan passed an audiology screening and, therefore, hearing problems can be ruled out. A more in-depth speech and language assessment finds that his muscle development is suitable for speech and that Ethan is using strategies such as pointing, grunting, or whining to get what he wants. His family is very good at anticipating his needs, and his older sister often talks for both of them. We hypothesize that Ethan's expressive communication skills are delayed because his current strategies work well enough for him, and he has less practice talking with people as a result
Intervention implementation	The interventionist works with Ethan's mother to increase opportunities for Ethan to use words to obtain what he wants. Ethan is offered choices of high interest activities, snacks, or other items, which are labeled for him verbally by mother and other family members. Ethan is praised for any attempt towards using words, which results in his obtaining the choice. Mother also helps to expand word phrases by modeling phrase speech, such as "You want the big, red truck." His mother is keeping a log of new words and phrases that Ethan uses, which are graphed weekly, to document his progress
Intervention evaluation	Six months later, Ethan's vocabulary has skyrocketed, making it difficult to count the number of spoken words. He is also beginning to use more 2–3 word phrases, make environmental sounds, and singing songs. The graph of new words and phrases shows that he is making progress with this intervention

Collaborative Problem Solving

The problem-solving process works best when developed with a team of individuals who are familiar with the child and her family. Members of the team might include providers from preschool, child protective services, primary care, and mental health, with each one helping to develop the plan that builds on the child and family's strengths to establish effective services and supports. Including a collaborative team in the problem-solving process has the potential to improve outcomes in a number of ways. For instance, through collaboration a child's providers may be able to more accurately define the presenting problem and generate hypotheses about why the problem is occurring. Through their coordinated efforts, this team will be more able to develop interventions that are linked to validated hypotheses as well as tailor them to the individual child and family.

As part of collaborative problem-solving process, establishing and maintaining rapport is essential. Initially building rapport may require a considerable amount of time and energy; however, the effectiveness and efficiency of the problem-solving process will improve as time goes on. For example, a caregiver must feel comfortable sharing sensitive information with the team such as whether or not they think they will be able to carry out the intervention as intended. If rapport has not been established, then the caregiver may agree to implement an intervention that they cannot carry out, and therefore, the benefit is lost. Developing and maintaining rapport involves active listening to the caregiver's perspective, developing shared goals, determining whether or not an intervention is acceptable and feasible to a caregiver, and sharing the importance of conducting the intervention as it is intended.

Conclusions

The prevention model is a notion which matches the level of care to a child's and family's needs. This model is frequently visually depicted by a pyramid, which outlines levels of support from least intensive to most intensive as based upon the needs of children and their families, and includes general education at the primary level which is expected to benefit most children and families, more focused guidance and support at the secondary level, aimed at children and families at higher risk, and extensive supports at the tertiary level, intended for those needing the most extensive support and intervention. The prevention model helps to guide the provision and funding of services and supports which are ultimately aimed to improve health and well-being of all children and their families. Within each level, the problem-solving process is used to pinpoint goals and objectives, and ensure that prevention and intervention efforts are appropriate and feasible. Lastly, data collection determines how well the intervention is working.

Assess Your Knowledge

1. Sandy enrolled in a group parent training class because her daughter Jenny has been throwing tantrums. Jenny has never been diagnosed with a disability, but recently has been engaging in more frequent tantrums. The group parent training class in which Sandy is enrolled fits best with which level of prevention?

   a. Primary
   b. Secondary

    c. Tertiary

    d. Problem solving

2. You have determined that the behavior of greatest concern with Kelly is hitting other children. You have determined that she does this three times more than her peers do. You have determined that the most likely reason for her behavior is that she does not have the skills to communicate her wants and need, which in turn leads to her hitting others. Using the problem-solving model, what would be your next step?

    a. Monitor the effects of your intervention

    b. Implement an intervention to teach Kelly communication skills

    c. Implement an intervention where you punish Kelly for hitting

    d. Identify the problem

3. Sophia's mother states that her daughter is behind in her motor skills. If you are following the problem-solving process what is your next step?

    a. Enroll Sophia in physical therapy

    b. Observe Sophia on the playground

    c. Gather information about Sophia's motor skills and compare this to established norms

    d. Send Sophia for evaluation by a specialist

4. Spencer was born 9 weeks premature and has experienced multiple developmental delays and difficulties in his early years (i.e., heart problems, feeding difficulties). Since Spencer has a number of needs, he receives an IFSP to promote his growth and development. This type of prevention strategy falls into what category?

    a. Primary

    b. Secondary

    c. Tertiary

    d. Problem solving

5. During what step of the problem-solving process should a team determine how they will measure the intervention's effects?

    a. Problem Identification

    b. Problem Analysis

    c. Intervention Implementation

    d. Intervention Evaluation

6. Effective prevention strategies at the secondary level should only be required by what percent of families?

    a. 75–85 %

    b. 45–65 %

    c. 15–25 %

    d. 5–15 %

7. Jessica is driving when she hears an ad for the "Let's Move" which provides information about improving nutrition and increasing activity so that individuals maintain a healthy weight. This campaign falls into what prevention tier?

    a. Primary
    b. Secondary
    c. Tertiary
    d. Problem solving

8. In the Intervention Implementation step, it is important to:

    a. Gather more information about the problem
    b. Evaluate the validity of each possible cause for the problem
    c. Examine the gap in skills between the children and their peers
    d. Determine who will implement the intervention and how long it will be tried

9. As the level of tiered services increases, what changes occur to progress monitoring?

    a. The frequency of progress monitoring increases
    b. Progress monitoring tools cost more
    c. The frequency of progress monitoring stays the same
    d. The frequency of progress monitoring decreases

10. If Ethan was not responding to the intervention conducted at home with his mother, what should the practitioner's next steps be?

    a. Continue the intervention
    b. Enroll Ethan's mother in a parenting class
    c. Implement a brand new intervention
    d. Recycle back through the problem-solving steps to generate a new intervention

Assess Your Knowledge Answers
1) b   2) b   3) c   4) c   5) c   6) d   7) a   8) d   9) a   10) d

Chapter 4
Screening Techniques

Abstract Child development involves the maturation and integration of an array of physical and cognitive functions. Although typical development occurs in a predictable sequence, there is also significant variability in rates of typical development. Screening techniques, such as standardized rating scales and observational tools, allow professionals to efficiently and accurately identify children who may be at risk for developmental delays or a developmental disorder. This chapter describes the benefits and limitations of developmental screeners in general and reviews a number of the screeners available to early childhood professionals.

Keywords Domains of development • Adaptive functioning • Communication skills • Motor development • Cognitive skills • Social/emotional development • Early identification • Screening • Assessment • Sensitivity • Specificity

Typical child development occurs in a predictable sequence marked by developmental milestones (Center for Disease Control and Prevention, 2011). Developmental milestones, such as taking a first step or saying a first word, are physical and behavioral signs of maturation that most children demonstrate within a certain window of time. The range for milestones can vary widely. For example, walking between 9 and 18 months is considered to reflect normal development. Milestones are achieved sequentially, where a child will first sit, then stand, walk, and run; but rates of development can vary significantly. For example, a baby might be very quiet and rarely make sounds or say words until her second birthday, and suddenly, she may not stop talking. For our convenience, developmental milestones are often categorized according to domains of development as if each were separate, when in fact they are all interrelated. These domains include (1) adaptive, (2) communication, (3) motor, (4) cognitive, and (5) social/emotional functioning and are described next.

K.H. Armstrong et al., *Evidence-Based Interventions for Children with Challenging Behavior*, DOI 10.1007/978-1-4614-7807-2_4,
© Springer Science+Business Media New York 2014

1. *Adaptive functioning,* also called self-help or independent skills, refers to skills, which help a child adapt to an environment or function independently. Early adaptive skills might include drinking from a cup or feeding oneself, while later skills include toilet training and dressing.
2. *Communication* milestones involve speaking, using and understanding body language and gestures, and understanding what others say. Early milestones include interest in sounds and words, while later milestones progress to describing play, answering questions, and engaging in conversations.
3. *Motor* skill milestones encompass maneuvering fingers and hands (fine motor skills) and large muscles movements of the arms and legs (gross motor skills). Examples of important motor early milestones are sitting independently and picking up small objects, while later milestones involve more complex skills such as running, navigating stairs, kicking a ball, or holding a crayon correctly.
4. *Cognitive* development milestones describe thinking skills, such as problem solving, maintaining attention, and understanding concepts. Early cognitive milestones involve exploration of objects with hands and mouth, while later skills include sorting objects by color, shape, and size.
5. *Social/emotional* development milestones describe emotions, interactions with others, and demonstration of feelings. Early social/emotional milestones include smiling at caregivers, while later milestones include playing with others, taking turns, and sharing.

For additional information on developmental milestones please refer to Web sites maintained by the American Academy of Pediatrics (AAP) (http://www.healthychildren.org/english/ages-stages/Pages/default.aspx; AAP, 2012) and the Center of Disease Control and Prevention (CDC) (http://www.cdc.gov/ncbddd/actearly/milestones/index.html; CDC, 2012).

The AAP recommends developmental surveillance at every Well-Child Visit and developmental screening using formal, validated tools at the 9, 18, 24, and 30 months Well-Child Visit or whenever a parent or provider concern is expressed (AAP, 2006). The AAP reports that 15–20 % of all visits to the pediatrician's office are developmental or behavioral in nature and 80 % of the parents' concerns regarding development are accurate. Therefore, early childhood professionals can anticipate having parents share developmental concerns with them, and these concerns should be considered as important sources of information. The following sections outline screening methods that may be useful to early childhood professionals.

Screening entails the administration of brief, standardized assessments to identify children who *may* have developmental delays (CDC, 2008). Screening tools can be categorized as general developmental screeners that cover all behavioral domains, or may be targeted screens which focus on one area of development. General screens can be completed by caregivers in offices or at home, or may be professionally administered by a trained professional.

When the results of the periodic screening tool are normal, an early childhood professional can inform the parents that their child's development is progressing well and continue with other aspects of the preventive visit. Normal screening results provide an opportunity to focus on developmental promotion. However, if screening results are concerning, the child should be scheduled for appropriate developmental evaluations as quickly as possible. This follow-up evaluation is aimed at identifying the specific developmental disorder(s) or delay(s) affecting the child, thus providing further prognostic information and allowing prompt initiation of specific and appropriate early childhood interventions.

Two broad techniques may be selected for the screening process: rating scales and observation. Rating scale screeners rely on caregiver reports of a child's behavior, and may be completed by the caregiver independently or through an interview between the examiner and the caregiver. Caregiver completed screening tools are an economical way to collect information about development, and in most cases, parents are excellent resources about their child's behavior. However, this type of screening may not be appropriate in certain instances, for example, with parents with mental retardation, parents with history of drug or alcohol problems, or families who do not speak English. Caregiver report measures should be easy to read, complete, score, and interpret. An example of a recommended caregiver report measure is *Ages and Stages Questionnaires*, which will be covered later in this chapter.

Observation screeners, on the other hand, require direct elicitation and observation of a child's skills by a trained professional. These screeners are more difficult and expensive to administer, as they require adherence to standardized administration procedures, and may not capture the skills a child possesses due to factors such as misunderstanding, lack of motivation or fatigue.

When selecting a screening tool, there are several factors to take into account. Technical adequacy refers to the psychometric properties of an instrument, and includes an examination of the instrument's validity and reliability. Thus, the screener should measure what it is intended to measure (validity), and perform consistently (reliability) over time. Secondly, the test floors and item gradients need to be considered, especially in the case of very young or delayed children. This means there must be enough early items so that a child at-risk can be identified, and enough incremental items to document even small gains in progress. Constructive validity refers to the degree to which the screening tool measures a construct of interest. This means that the tool should screen for the problem of concern, for example, if communication milestones are a worry, the tool should assess communication skills. Lastly, predictive validity refers to the assumption that screeners accurately and predictably identify concerns.

And practically, the screening tool is meant to be brief (no longer than 30 min), easy to administer and score, and of low cost. The objective for screening is to quickly and accurately identify children in need of more intensive assessment. The primary purpose of a screening tool is to identify children at-risk, in order to refer them for more comprehensive assessment and possible services. The utility of a screening tool is often referred to as its hit rate, or its success in identifying children who do or do not need additional assessment.

Screening outcomes are described as *true positives, false negatives, false positives, and true negatives*. A true positive correctly identifies child at-risk, who will need additional assessment. A false negative fails to identify a child at-risk, who

Table 4.1 Formula to calculate sensitivity and specificity of screening tool

Developmental delay			
	Present	Absent	
+	a (true positive)	b (false positive)	$a+b$
−	c (false negative)	d (true negative)	$c+d$
	$a+c$	$b+d$	$a+b+c+d$

Table 4.2 Practice example calculating sensitivity and specificity of a screening tool

Developmental delay			
	Present	Absent	
+	a (80)	b (10)	$a+b=90$
−	c (10)	d (50)	$c+d=60$
	$a+c=90$	$b+d=60$	$a+b+c+d=150$

Sensitivity = 80/90 = 89 %
Specificity = 50/60 = 83 %

should receive additional assessment. A false positive identifies risk when it is no risk, and a true negative correctly identifies children who do not need additional assessment. Thus, one wants to select a screening tool which maximizes true positives and true negatives.

Two additional terms are used to describe how well the screening tool performs: Sensitivity and Specificity. Sensitivity refers to the proportion of children with developmental delays who are detected by the screener (true positives) and if the tool has higher sensitivity, you are better able to rule out the delay. Specificity refers to the proportion of children without developmental delay who are not identified with delay by the screener (true negative). High specificity will rule in the delay.

Table 4.1 represents screening results for four possible groups of children, labeled a, b, c, d. Sensitivity is calculated as $a/(a+c)$. Specificity is calculated as $d/(b+d)$. We want to find tools which achieve sensitivity and specificity of greater than or equal to 80 %, to be able to say with confidence that we have a good *hit rate*.

Here is a practice example using the formula shown above in selecting a new screener. You will screen 150 2-year-old children (you already know whether or not they have developmental delays). Eighty children with delays screen positive for a delay. Ten children with a delay are not picked up by the screener, and screen negative. Another ten children without delay are incorrectly identified by the screener with a delay. And 50 children without delay are correctly screened as negative or no delay. Table 4.2 graphically depicts these numbers.

Using this example, your calculations tell you that 89 % of children with developmental delay screen positive with the screening tool, and 83 % of children who do not have a delay screen negative. The cutoff score used to indicate acceptable sensitivity and specificity is 80 % or higher. Thus you would conclude that this tool does an adequate job in identifying children who should be referred for additional assessment, and does not overidentify delays in those without delays.

Table 4.3 Ages and Stages Questionnaires-Third Edition (ASQ-3; Bricker & Squires, 2009)

Domain(s):	Communication, motor skills, cognitive development, social/emotional development	For:	Children 1–66 months of age
Type:	Rating scale	Length:	10–15 min to administer 2–3 min to score
Description:	ASQ-3 consists of 21 age-specific questionnaires that allow for developmental screening at different intervals, such as at the recommended 9-, 18-, and 24- or 30- month Well-Child Visits. Parents respond *Yes*, *Sometimes*, or *Not Yet* to each item		
Strengths:	Requires minimal training; reproducible materials; easy to read items (Hanig, 2012); available in several languages	Limitations:	Validity data are somewhat weak (Hanig, 2012)
Web site:	http://www.agesandstages.com/		

Table 4.4 Ages and Stages Questionnaire: Social Emotional (ASQ-SE; Squires, Bricker, Twombly, & Yockelson, 2001)

Domain(s):	Social/emotional (i.e., self-regulation, compliance, adaptive behaviors, communication, affect, autonomy, and social interactions)	For:	Children 3–66 months of age
Type:	Rating scale	Length:	10–15 min to administer; 2–3 to score
Description:	ASQ-SE screens for social-emotional problems with eight different questionnaires each covering 3 month intervals		
Strengths:	Available in Spanish; easy to use and understand (Vacca, 2005)	Limitations:	Generalizability of scores across gender, race, and ethnicity is unknown (Vacca, 2012)
Web site:	http://www.agesandstages.com/		

Several screeners are available for use with young children that are quick and simple to administer and score, as well as reliable and valid for identifying developmental delays. Screener descriptions, domains assessed, appropriate age groups for use, length of time for administration and scoring, as well as the strengths and limitations of the screening tools are provided within each table (Tables 4.3, 4.4, 4.5, 4.6, 4.7, 4.8, 4.9, 4.10, 4.11, and 4.12).

Table 4.5 Battelle Developmental Inventory-Second Edition screening test (BDIST; Newborg, 2005)

Domain(s):	Social/emotional, adaptive functioning, motor skills, communication, and cognitive development	For:	Children from birth to 7 years 11 months of age
Type:	Observation and direct elicitation of skills	Length:	10–30 min
Description:	Consists of 100 items from the full battery assessment and results of this screening indicate whether or not the full battery should be administered		
Strengths:	Available in other languages; flexible administrative procedures (Athanasiou, 2007)	Limitations:	Scoring criteria of some items are ambiguous (Athanasiou, 2007)
Web site:	http://www.riverpub.com/products/bdi2/details.html		

Table 4.6 Bayley Infant Neurodevelopmental Screener (BINS; Aylward, 1995)

Domain(s):	Basic neurological functions (i.e., auditory and visual receptive functions, verbal and motor expressive functions, and cognitive processes)	For:	Children 3–24 months of age
Type:	Observation and direct elicitation of skills	Length:	10–15 min to administer 3 min to score
Description:	The BINS contains selected items from the Bayley Scales of Infant Development-Second Edition (BSID-II) and neurological assessments		
Strengths:	Exceptionally clear and concise administrative instructions; kit provides all necessary materials; works well in setting where many infants have to be screened daily (Benish, 2007)	Limitations:	A structured observation and clinical interview would likely be just as effective as the BINS in a setting with fewer infants (Benish, 2007)
Web site:	http://www.pearsonassessments.com/HAIWEB/Cultures/en-us/Productdetail. htm?Pid=015-8028-708&Mode=summary		

Table 4.7 Brief Infant-Toddler Social and Emotional Assessment (BITSEA; Briggs-Gowan & Carter, 2006)

Domain(s):	Social-emotional (i.e., externalizing, internalizing, dysregulation, and competence)	For:	Children 12–35 months of age
Type:	Rating scale	Length:	7–10 min to administer
Description:	The BITSEA is a 42-item Parent Form that can be completed quickly to screen for social-emotional problems in children. The infant-toddler social and emotional assessment (ITSEA) is designed to be used subsequently		
Strengths:	Requires minimal training; available in Spanish; provides a childcare form to allow for multiple raters; computer scoring	Limitations:	Little information in the manual about empirical support for the reliability and validity of scores from the childcare form (Konold, 2007)
Web site:	http://www.pearsonassessments.com/HAIWEB/Cultures/en-us/Productdetail. htm?Pid=015-8007-352&Mode=summary		

Table 4.8 Brigance Early Childhood Screens (Brigance & Glascoe, 2010)

Domain(s):	Communication, motor, adaptive functioning, social/emotional, and cognitive	For:	For children 0–60 months of age
Type:	Observation and direct elicitation of skills	Length:	10–15 min to administer
Description:	These early childhood screens, which are part of the comprehensive Brigance early childhood system, can identify both learning delays and giftedness. Three screens are available, with one specifically for children 0–35 months of age		
Strengths:	Free online training	Limitations:	Not yet reviewed
Web site:	http://www.curriculumassociates.com/products/detail.aspx?title=brigec-screens&topic=CEC0		

Table 4.9 Communication and Symbolic Behavior Scales Developmental Profile (CSBS DP) infant/toddler checklist (Wetherby & Prizant, 2002)

Domain(s):	Communication	For:	Children 6–24 months of age
Type:	Rating scale	Length:	5–10 min
Description:	This instrument is composed of 24 multiple choice items grouped into social, speech, and symbolic composite scores		
Strengths:	Free to download online	Limitations:	Lack of national norms and may not be appropriate for use with minority and low socioeconomic populations (Carey, 2012)
Web site:	http://firstwords.fsu.edu/index.php/early-identification-of-communication-delays		

Table 4.10 Modified Checklist for Autism in Toddlers (M-CHAT; Robins, Fein, & Barton, 1999)

Domain(s):	Screener for autism spectrum disorder	For:	Children 16–30 months of age
Type:	Rating scale	Length:	5–7 min to administer Under 2 min to score
Description:	Parents complete a 23-item form with *Yes* and *No* responses to assess characteristics of an autism spectrum disorder		
Strengths:	Available for free online, available in multiple languages	Limitations:	High false-positive rate
Web site:	http://www2.gsu.edu/~psydlr/Diana_L._Robins,_Ph.D..html		

Table 4.11 Parents' Evaluation of Developmental Status (PEDS; Glascoe, 2010)

Domain(s):	Cognitive development, communication, motor skills, social/emotional development, adaptive functioning	For:	Children from birth to 7 years and 11 months of age
Type:	Rating scale	Length:	2 min to administer and score
Description:	This ten-item screener elicits parent concerns across the different developmental domains		
Strengths:	Brief, inexpensive easy to administer and score, ideal for use by healthcare providers (Bischoff, 2012; Roberts, 2012)	Limitations:	None identified in the independent review
Web site:	http://www.pedstest.com		

Table 4.12 PEDS: Developmental Milestones (PEDS:DM; Glascoe, 2008)

Domain(s):	Motor skills, communication, adaptive functioning, social/emotional development	For:	Children from birth to 7 years and 11 months of age
Type:	Rating scale	Length:	5 min to administer 1 min to score
Description:	PEDS:DM ranges from 6 to 8 items and is best used in combination with the PEDS but it can also be used alone		
Strengths:	Not yet reviewed	Limitations:	Not yet reviewed
Web site:	http://www.pedstest.com		

Conclusions

In sum, screeners are important tools for early intervention professionals because they provide valuable information about a child's development. Screening information can be helpful towards identifying concerns and determining if more in-depth assessment and intervention is needed. If screener results suggest that there may be a developmental delay then a comprehensive evaluation should follow. However, not all screening tools are equally useful. In selecting a screening tool, one should make sure that the tool is able to assess the problem, has adequate specificity and sensitivity, is brief to administer, easy to score, is useful in providing information about important and meaningful skills, and can be used repeatedly on a frequent basis (Ikeda, Neessen, & Witt, 2008).

Assess Your Knowledge

1. Please list and describe the five domains used to categorize developmental milestones.

   a.

   b.

   c.

   d.

   e.

2. What is the advantage of using a screening tool with young children?

   a. To obtain comprehensive evaluation results
   b. To diagnose a child as having a developmental delay
   c. To determine if more in-depth evaluation is needed to identify a developmental delay
   d. Both a and b

3. True or False: Screeners should be able to assess the identified problem, specific and sensitive, brief to administer and score, useful in providing information about important and meaningful skills, and be used repeatedly on a frequent basis.
4. What are the two broad techniques used for screening?

   a.
   b.

5. If screener results suggest that there may be a developmental delay then what should be done next?
6. Calculate the following rates of sensitivity and specificity for screening tool A and decide whether this tool will do an adequate job in screening children for developmental delay:200 children are screened with screening tool A for developmental delay. It identifies 100 as true positives, 20 children as true negatives, 20 children as false positives, and 60 children as false negatives.

   a. Sensitivity
   b. Specificity

Assess Your Knowledge Answers
1) adaptive, communication, cognition, motor, social/emotional   2) c   3) True
4) observational, rating   5) Refer   6) Sensitivity = 83 %; Specificity = 75 %

Chapter 5
Evidence-Based Practices with Children and Their Caregivers

Abstract When delivering services to children and their caregivers, it is important for early intervention professionals to integrate their clinical expertise, the family's values, and the best research evidence into selecting strategies to improve developmental outcomes. Referred to as evidence-based practice, this process enhances both optimal outcomes and quality of life by utilizing interventions that have been documented through systematic research efforts.

Keywords Evidence-based practice • Clinical expertise • PICO • Efficacy • Case studies • Case control studies • Cohort studies • Randomized control trial • Systematic review • Meta-analysis • Treatment and control group • Validity • Confidence intervals • *P* value • Risks and benefits

Evidence-based practice (EBP) refers to a process in which scientifically supported interventions are selected to improve outcomes and/or reduce other complications that may otherwise impede healthy development. First described by medicine, EBP was described as "the conscientious, explicit, and judicious use of current best evidence in making decisions about the care of an individual patient" (Sackett et al., 1996, p. 71). EBP integrates the provider's clinical expertise, patient values, and the best research evidence into the intervention process. Clinical expertise refers to the early intervention professional's cumulated experience, education, and skills. The child's caregivers bring their own personal and unique preferences, concerns, and values. And, the best evidence for the intervention is documented through carefully conducted and published research studies.

PICO is an acronym that helps practitioners frame a specific clinical question about which evidence will be sought. PICO stands for patient population or problem, Intervention, Comparison and Outcome. In thinking about the "P," patient population or problem, the key problems and characteristic of the child and family are described, which might be relevant in selecting the intervention. This might

Table 5.1 Examples of PICO process to describe parenting programs

Population	Intervention	Comparison	Outcome
All caregivers and children ages 6 months to 5 years (primary prevention)	Reach Out and Read	• Online training • Cohort studies	• Increased receptive vocabulary • Increased frequency in reading activities
Caregivers of 18-month–5-year-old children, concerned with their child's behavior (secondary prevention)	Helping Our Toddlers, Developing Our Children's Skills	• Manualized program • Cohort and case studies	• Reduction in child behavior problems • Increase in caregiver knowledge and skills
Children with autism spectrum disorders, ages 18 months to 8 years (tertiary prevention)	Lovaas Applied Behavior Analysis (ABA)	• Manualized program • Two Cohort studies	• Improvements in IQ, language, and functional skills

include the primary referral problem, coexisting conditions, age, sex, or race. The "I" or intervention is the main intervention that one is considering in order to achieve certain goals. The "C" refers to how well the selected intervention compares to other interventions as well as to whether the information is specific enough to really describe what to do with the child and their caregivers. And, "O" refers to the outcome of interest, which could be both specific and functional. An example of the PICO process as used to address children presenting in well-child visits, children presenting with challenging behavior, and children with autism spectrum disorders is described in the Table 5.1.

To become recognized as evidence-based, a program must be documented through careful research and evaluation studies using rigorous scientific methods and procedures. This ensures that the interventions do more good than harm and are worth the efforts and costs of using them (Chorpita, 2003). There are many types of studies which are conducted in order to provide evidence of the intervention, sometimes referred to as the hierarchy of study design, and are used to document the evolution of the research literature. Starting first with ideas, these interventions are tested more and more rigorously in order to document their efficacy and safety. Types of studies going from lowest to highest level of design include Case Studies, Case Control Studies, Cohort Studies, Randomized Control Trial, Systematic Review, and Meta-analysis and are briefly described below:

Case studies consist of reports on the intervention used with a single individual or individuals, but there are no control groups with which to compare outcomes. Thus, case studies are not considered to have statistical validity.

Case control studies include studies in which individuals with a certain condition are compared with other people who do not have that condition. Often records such as medical or school reports are reviewed for data. This type of study is considered to be observational and not as reliable as randomized control studies.

Randomized control studies are studies in which individuals are randomly assigned to a treatment or control group, and their outcomes are documented and compared. This type of design helps to provide sound evidence of cause and effect.

Systematic reviews are conducted to review studies on a certain topic, in order to answer specific questions. The selected studies must have sound methodology in order to be included in the review.

Meta-analysis is a statistical method which is used to combine the results from several valid studies on a particular intervention and report it as if it were one study.

Early intervention providers seeking to engage in evidence-based practice must keep current with their professional literature, in order to know which interventions are the best suited for the children and families that they serve. There are three basic questions that need to be answered in order to evaluate any study:

1. Are the results of the study valid?
2. What are the results?
3. Will the results help in caring for my client(s)?

Validity refers to truthfulness or soundness of the study methodology. Some key aspects that support the validity of a study is the similarity of the treatment and control groups before the intervention, random assignment of individuals to treatment or control groups, and follow-up on the individuals who completed the study.

The results or outcomes of the study should also be presented in terms of statistical significance. Confidence intervals are a measure of the precision of a study, meaning the chance for error if the study were repeated again. Smaller intervals show greater precision. *P* value refers to the probability that any outcome would have arisen by chance. The smaller the *P* value, the higher the significance.

Lastly, it is important to make sure that the intervention selected is suitable for your client (s). First your client(s) must be comparable to the study participants to make sure that this is a good match. Second, make sure that published research supports the outcomes that you hope to attain. Programs can be described as *Possibly Efficacious* or *Well-Established* depending upon the degree of research evidence supporting their outcomes. *Possibly* Efficacious programs should include published case studies and case control studies, while well-established programs are supported by randomized control trials.

There are numerous advantages to EBP, namely that it encourages professionals to stay current and use the most appropriate information available in assisting their clients. In recent years, professional organizations such as the American Psychological Association (APA), the American Occupational Therapy Association, the American Nurses Association, and the American Physical Therapy Association have strongly encouraged their members to engage in EBP. As such, we have elected to employ the scheme proposed by Chambless and Hollon (1998) and APA Division 12 Task Force on Psychological Interventions which may be used to determine when a psychological treatment for a specific problem may be considered well established in efficacy or possibly efficacious. Well-established treatments include those in which benefits to clients have been replicated by at least one independent research team(s). Possibly efficacious includes interventions that have published evaluation data that document improved outcomes for children and families but have not been replicated by independent teams.

The remainder of this chapter will review programs appropriate for the early childhood years that have documented effectiveness for the individuals and families targeted and are broadly grouped into two categories: (1) parent/child programs, and (2) child/classroom programs. Within each of these categories, programs are discussed according to their designation within the prevention model, i.e., primary, secondary, or tertiary. Details including target population, presentation, theoretical background, time and training requirements, costs, and empirical support will be covered in the narratives. Summary tables of each of the reviewed programs are found at the introduction of each section, with comparison ratings of Possibly Efficacious or Well-Established (Table 5.2). However, keep in mind that research efforts are continuous and over time new evidence may emerge that strengthens or challenges these approaches for certain populations or within certain circumstances.

Parent/Child Programs: Primary Prevention

Reach Out and Read (ROR) was the only primary prevention program identified as part of this review. ROR will be described below.

Reach Out and Read

Distinguishing Features

ROR can be distinguished from other programs by settings where it is put in place (primary care) and the universal approach it takes to ensuring all children get literacy exposure during the early years of development. ROR is usually implemented in pediatricians' offices where children would go to receive *well-child visits*. There are three separate components to the ROR program: (1) encouraging parents to read with their children and instructing parents on how this can be done, (2) providing every parent of a child 6 months to 5 years old with an age-appropriate book, and (3) having volunteer readers or providing early literacy materials in the waiting room.

Theoretical Grounding

ROR has developed out of research that documents the importance of exposing children to literacy prior to entering formal schooling. Additionally, the program also addresses research indicating that certain groups of families (low-income, minority, and nonnative English speakers) are difficult to reach and engage in early intervention practices (Zuckerman, 2009).

Table 5.2 Summary of parent/child programs using PICO process

	Population	Intervention	Comparison	Outcome
Primary prevention program				
Reach Out and Read	6 months to 5 years	Literacy exposure in well-child visits	Possibly efficacious	Higher receptive vocabulary; greater frequency of reading activities
Secondary prevention programs				
Helping Our Toddlers Developing Our Children's Skills	18–60 months	Behavioral parent training	Possibly efficacious	Decreased child behavior problems; Improved parenting skills; Increased engagement of fathers and Spanish speakers
Incredible Years	Birth–12 years	Behavioral parent training	Well-established	Decreased child behavior problems; Improved parenting skills; works well with low-income, racially and ethnically diverse families
Nurse-Family Partnership	Low-income mothers, prenatal-2 years	Preventive health care, positive parenting, self-sufficiency	Well-established	Improved health practices and parenting skills; long-term improvements in child outcomes
Parents are Teachers	Low-income families, birth-5 years	School readiness, positive parenting practices	Possibly efficacious	Improved health and school readiness, improved parenting practices
Tertiary prevention programs				
Helping the Noncompliant Child	3–8 years	Improved parenting skills and child behavior/compliance	Well-established	More compliance to adult direction, and improved parenting skills
Lovaas Applied Behavior Analysis	18 months to 8 years	Increased communication and functional skills for children with autism spectrum disorder (ASD)	Well-established	Improvement in communication, adaptive skills, increased IQ scores in older children
Parent–Child Interaction Therapy	2.5–7 years	Improved parenting skills and child behavior/compliance	Well-established	More compliance to adult direction, and improved parenting skills
Trauma-Focused Cognitive Behavior Therapy	3–17 years	Reduced PTSD symptoms; improved problem solving and coping skills	Well-established	Fewer PTSD symptoms, improved parenting skills
Multitiered programs				
Triple P	Birth-18 years	Create healthy families	Possibly efficacious	Reduced child behavior problems and parenting stress; improved parent mental health and relationships

Focus

The focus of ROR is to increase young children's exposure to print and improve the home literacy environment through providing books and parent instruction. ROR specifically targets children who are at risk for not being exposed to reading early in life. Children between the ages of 6 months and 5 years old are eligible to participate in this program.

Time Requirements

ROR occurs during regularly scheduled Well-Child Visit (WCV). The program begins with volunteer readers interacting with parents in the waiting room to model reading strategies or through the provision of information via pamphlets/fact sheets. As part of the physical exam, the physician or nurse suggests books and strategies that the caregiver may use to promote reading. This discussion may extend the appointment by a few minutes, but in general, the program does not require any time more than a typical WCV. The program targets infants and children from age 6 months to 5 years.

Child Participation

Children participate in the intervention with their parents by attending the doctor's visits and engaging in reading activities with the waiting room volunteer. Children also engage in the intervention after their doctor's visit is completed by reading with their parents.

Progress Monitoring Tools

There are no specific tools used with ROR to track child progress or frequency of parent–child reading activities. Books are recommended based upon developmental milestones.

Training Requirements/Cost

Information about ROR training is available through the website www.reachoutandread.org. Depending upon the number of physicians, nurses and other staff, and the location, a variety of training options are available. This includes a live training with an ROR Trainer and Provider, an online class for CME credit, or a simple premade presentation for the clinic staff. Training costs include copies of materials.

Materials

To reduce costs, many clinics have arranged for book donations and community volunteers through the ROR website. New books are available from the ROR organization for the cost of about $2.75 per book. Many materials (handouts, milestone fact sheets) are available from www.reachoutandread.org after providers register with this nonprofit organization. In addition, educators and parents can access the website for book lists, a sheet of milestones for literacy, and more information about reading to young children and the impact it can have.

Empirical Support

ROR has been investigated in 14 studies that have been published in the research literature and meets criteria for a *Possibly Efficacious* intervention program. Most studies included participants with low socio-economic backgrounds and/or minority racial and ethnic backgrounds. Parents who were in an ROR program have been shown to improve the frequency of engaging in reading-related activities (Golova, Alario, Vivier, Rodriguez, & High, 1999; High, Hopman, LaGasse, & Linn, 1998; High, LaGasse, Becker, Ahlgren, & Gardner, 2000; Mendelsohn et al., 2001; Needleman, Toker, Dreyer, Klass, & Mendelsohn, 2005; Sanders, Gershon, Huffman, & Mendoza, 2000; Silverstein, Iverson, & Lozano, 2002; Weitzman, Roy, Walls, & Tomlin, 2004). Additionally, receiving ROR has been shown to increase reports that children list reading as a favorite activity (High et al., 1998, 2000; Silverstein et al., 2002; Theriot et al., 2003; Weitzman et al., 2004). Finally, three studies have examined changes in child vocabulary skills and found that in general, exposure to the ROR program is related to higher receptive vocabulary (Mendelsohn et al., 2001; Sharif, Rieber, & Ozuah, 2002; Theriot et al., 2003).

Prevention Model Tier

ROR is considered a tier 1 prevention program since it is designed to be used with *all* children as a way to ensure exposure to reading and literacy early in life. This intervention is not time-intensive, has little cost associated with it, and is delivered in the same manner to all children.

Parent/Child Programs: Secondary Prevention

A review of secondary prevention programs identified four programs: *Helping Our Toddlers, Developing our Children's Skills, Incredible Years, Nurse-Family Partnerships, and Parents as Teachers.*

Helping Our Toddlers, Developing Our Children's Skills (HOT DOCS)

Distinguishing Features

Helping Our Toddlers, Developing Our Children's Skills (HOT DOCS; Armstrong, Lilly, Agazzi, & Williams, 2010) is a parenting program that was developed at the University of South Florida Department of Pediatrics. It can be distinguished from other parenting programs since it helps parents and caregivers apply a problem-solving model to understand and address challenging behaviors. HOT DOCS may be used in a group setting or with individual families (Curtiss, Armstrong, & Lilly, 2008). Information is conveyed through live and video-taped instruction, role playing, modeling, and practice exercises. The program is available in English and Spanish (Armstrong, Agazzi, Childres, & Lilly, 2012).

Theoretical Grounding

HOT DOCS is grounded in social learning, developmental, and attachment theories and combines behavioral approaches to learning within nurturing and responsive relationships (Armstrong, Hornbeck, Beam, Mack, & Popkave, 2006). The program also takes an ecological approach, by encouraging multiple caregivers to attend the training so that handling of the child's behavior is consistent across settings. Through changing the caregiver's behavior and responsiveness to the child, the child's functioning can be improved.

Focus

HOT DOCS uses a problem-solving chart with parents and caregivers that helps them understand why problem behavior occurs, and how to develop strategies that reduce or eliminate problem behaviors while teaching more adaptive skills. The program has documented improvement for children who are between the ages of 18 months and 6 years old, but has been used successfully with children outside of that range who have developmental disabilities (Williams, Armstrong, Agazzi, & Bradley-Klug, 2010).

Time Requirements

With group implementation, HOT DOCS consists of seven 2½ hour meetings, while individual implementation can occur weekly as needed within home or daycare settings. Weekly homework assignments facilitate practice of new skills and include both a child-focused component and parent-focused component.

Child Participation

Children do not participate directly in the group parent training. With home visits, interactions between caregivers and children are observed, and feedback is offered. However, all homework activities are designed to improve interactions between parents and/or professional caregivers and their children.

Progress Monitoring Tools

Throughout the sessions, participants complete homework and progress monitoring activities which allow the trainer to determine the level of understanding they have achieved for skills presented in the previous lesson. These assignments also allow the trainer to provide individualized feedback on skills. The participants also complete a multiple choice test on the ideas central to HOT DOCS prior to attending and at the end of the last session to evaluate knowledge of content. Finally, the authors recommend that all participants complete a standardized behavior rating scale prior to beginning classes and after the final session.

Training Requirements/Cost

There are two options for becoming a HOT DOCS trainer. The first is to attend all sessions of a training as a participant, and then to co-teach an entire course with an experienced trainer. This route requires potential trainers to purchase the trainers manual which is included in the registration fee and participate in a group lead by a master HOT DOCS trainer. Another option is to have an experienced HOT DOCS trainer deliver an all-day Train-the-Trainers workshop which would allow all staff attending to begin delivering HOT DOCS to their clients. The cost for this is $1,500 plus the cost of travel and manuals for participants. For more information and prices go to http://health.usf.edu/medicine/pediatrics/child-dev-neuro/HOTDOCS.htm.

Materials

The materials for conducting HOT DOCS sessions include a trainer's manual which includes the training DVD, and a participant workbook ($30) for each adult participating in the group. Also, trainers must have some way of projecting the PowerPoint slides and videos used for teaching each session. In addition, the trainer should provide items for the "Special Play" activity which is assigned every week. These items include bubbles, books, crayons and coloring books, Play Doh, and balls, enough to give one to each participating family. A final item that participants receive is a laminated HOT DOCS chart which may be written on with a dry erase marker.

Empirical Support

Several published studies supporting the benefit of the HOT DOCS program make it a *Possibly Efficacious* treatment. Analyses indicate that parents perceived positive outcomes for themselves and their children after participating in the program regardless of caregivers' level of education and availability of social support, showed increases in child development knowledge and high levels of satisfaction with the program, and reductions in child behavior on standardized rating scales (Williams, 2007, 2009; Williams et al., 2010). The positive experience of participant fathers has been documented through focus group interviews which identified key strategies to increase male caregivers' participation in parent training (Salinas, Smith, & Armstrong, 2011). In addition, the HOT DOCS approach has been adapted for Hispanic caregivers and has been translated into Spanish (Agazzi et al., 2010). Results for a wait-list cohort study also showed improved behavioral functioning of the treatment group (Williams, Agazzi, & Armstrong, 2011). Lastly, implementation has been documented for its use with toddler feeding concerns (Childres, Shaffer-Hudkins, & Armstrong, in press; Curtiss et al., 2008) and for autism spectrum disorders.

Prevention Model Tier

HOT DOCS is considered to be a tier 2 prevention program since it is designed for caregivers of children who believe that their children exhibit high levels of challenging behavior and/or developmental delays and disabilities. The intervention may be provided in a group format, making it less expensive compared with programs that require individual attention for each parent and/or child. HOT DOCS may also be applied individually within a home setting, and thus adapts well to home-based early intervention (Curtiss et al., 2008).

Incredible Years

Distinguishing Features

Incredible Years Programs (IYP) can be distinguished from other parenting programs by the extensive use of videotape vignettes throughout all training series. IYP was developed by Carolyn Webster-Stratton in 1980 and has expanded from solely a parent training program into a set of programs addressing concerns by working with parents, teachers, and the children exhibiting noncompliant and aggressive behavior. The different subprograms can be separated by the age of the child (programs address concerns from birth to age 12) and areas of concern (some focus on school, others on home). The curriculum teaches skills to the participants through behaviorally based strategies that include video-taped vignettes, modeling, role-playing, group discussion, and homework.

Theoretical Grounding

IYP is grounded in the research on factors associated with early-onset of aggression and conduct problems and Albert Bandura's research on the impact of modeling to change behavior (Webster-Stratton & Reid, 2003). The overall approach for the training model is a social learning approach (Sampers, Anderson, Hartung, & Scambler, 2001).

Focus

The focus of the IYP is to increase the competencies of parents and teachers to use nonphysical discipline strategies in order to handle noncompliant and aggressive behavior and to promote appropriate child behavior.

Time Requirements

The time required to complete the different programs varies. The parenting programs can last from 13 to 28 weeks and sessions are usually held every week for 2 hours (Reid & Webster-Stratton, 2001).

Child Participation

Children do not participate in the intervention with their parents. However, IYP has a companion program for children called the Dina Dinosaur program which is available in classroom and small group format. More information on the child programs is available through the IYP website www.incredibleyears.com and in the "Child/Classroom" section in this chapter.

Progress Monitoring Tools

A number of tools are available on the IY website (www.incredibleyears.com) to track the progress of the child, parent, or teacher. Also included are a number of tools to assess the group leader's adherence to the training manual and the ratings of each session and the IY program overall.

Training Requirements/Cost

To maintain consistently high standards in how the training is delivered to parents, teachers, and children, the staff at IY require all group members to attend a 3-day workshop before delivering the intervention. These workshops are offered at a variety of locations around the nation. The Seattle workshops typically cost around $400. For more information visit the IY website at www.incredibleyears.com. In addition, it is possible for trainers to receive certification to provide training (certified group leader) and to train other providers (certified mentor or certified trainer) through additional workshops and materials.

In addition to these costs, trainers must purchase the materials for each program they wish to use. Programs range in cost depending on the number ordered and type (some saving occurs with bundling), but costs begin at $995 and increase. Also available are additional DVDs with vignettes and training sessions for providers, and materials to supplement IY sessions.

Materials

Essential materials include the items in the program package along with some method of showing them to families (TV & DVD player or computer & projector). Also, each participant requires a book and/or workbook.

Empirical Support

Incredible Years has a widely established research base with many rigorous research studies indicating its effectiveness with a variety of populations. The parent intervention for 2–8-year-olds has met criteria for a *Well-Established* evidence-based intervention (Chambless & Hollon, 1998). Most research has focused on the parent intervention, with the exception of very limited literature being found on the more recently developed Babies & Toddlers programs. The parenting programs have been found to work with parents of children who have developmental delays (McIntyre, 2008), low-income and urban populations (Gross et al., 2003), and with racially and ethnically diverse parents (Reid, Webster-Stratton, & Beauchaine, 2002). The program has also been found to be effective when provided entirely on the computer with activities and handouts to be completed independently (Taylor et al., 2008).

Prevention Model Tier

IYP is a secondary or tier 2 prevention program, as activities target parents of children who may be at risk for disruptive and noncompliant behavior problems, but do not necessarily carry a diagnosis. The program is provided in a group format and teaches skills that are intended to improve child functioning.

Nurse-Family Partnership

Distinguishing Features

The Nurse-Family Partnership (NFP) is a program which begins working with first-time mothers identified during the prenatal period and continues the relationship through the child's second birthday. NFP can also be distinguished from other programs since it can only be implemented with trained, registered nurses as the home-visitors. The program was originally developed by Dr. David Olds in the late 1970s as a solution to preventing the multitude of negative outcomes for children growing up in urban environments. An initial focus was to prevent child abuse and neglect by providing support and knowledge to families. The focus has now expanded to improving multiple areas of a family's life (relationships, economic, health, etc.). The program is implemented in certain areas around the country by local agencies which provide home-visiting nurses with supervision and collect and analyze data regarding effectiveness of NFP locally and examine fidelity to the intervention plan.

Theoretical Grounding

NFP pulls from three primary theories within the developmental psychology literature. The first is Bandura's self-efficacy theory which holds that people are more likely to engage in a behavior if they believe they can successfully complete the behavior and a desired outcome will result. A second influence is Bronfenbrenner's ecological theory, a view that where families live and the relationships that a family has with other people influences how parents care for their children. NFP is also grounded in Bowlby's attachment theory in that NFP focuses on enhancing parents' sensitive and responsive parenting behaviors in order to strengthen a bond between parents and child and to improve the likelihood that children will grow up and establish healthy relationships with others.

Focus

The focus of NFP is to improve child development by (1) improving pregnancy outcomes for first-time mothers by exposing them to good preventive health practices and ensuring thorough prenatal care, (2) helping parents provide responsible and competent care, and (3) improving the home environment by helping parents become economically self-sufficient, plan future pregnancies, and continue their education or find work.

Time Requirements

The program typically works with families during their first trimester through the child's second birthday, lasting a total of 30 months. The visits are scheduled weekly for the first month a mother is enrolled and then they occur bi-weekly until the child is born. After the child is born, visits occur weekly for the first 6 weeks and then occur bi-weekly until the child is 20 months old. The last four visits occur once a month until the child is 2 years of age.

Child Participation

Children participate in activities with the nurse during the visit.

Progress Monitoring Tools

Data is collected at each NFP visit and is entered into a national data-base for analysis. This is to ensure that the fidelity of NFP session is maintained at the same level as the clinical trials. These tools appear to be standard across all agencies, but none are readily available to the public.

Training Requirements/Cost

The program does require training for registered nurses prior to working with families. It is suggested that nurses have previous experience in maternal or child health, behavioral health nursing, pediatrics, or other related fields. The core NFP training is offered in both face-to-face and distance learning opportunities. Nurses also meet regularly with a supervisor at their local agency to review family progress and address any concerns within the nurse-mother relationship. In addition, a manual provides guidance for what topics to be covered in each home session with parents. The manual allows for some flexibility in providing services to families. No cost data were available from the program's website (www.nursefamilypartnership.org).

Materials

Once a nurse becomes employed by a local agency, all materials are provided. To find a local agency, visit the program's website at www.nursefamilypartnership.org.

Empirical Support

The NFP has received extensive research support over the last 30 years of implementation. It meets criteria for a *Well-Established* intervention program. Through three randomized controlled trials conducted with families of Hispanic, African-American, and Caucasian backgrounds in rural and urban communities, the program continues to generate positive outcomes (Kitzman et al., 1997; Olds,

Henderson, & Kitzman, 1994; Olds et al., 2002). Extensive follow-up on the participants who were in the trials has proven that the NFP improves outcomes for mothers in multiple domains (e.g., improved prenatal health, reduce economic dependence on federal aid, reduce substance abuse problems and arrests) and child development outcomes have also shown improvement in many areas as a result of the program (e.g., increased school readiness, fewer arrests at age 15, fewer child injuries, and reduced abuse of substances; Eckenrode et al., 2000, 2010; Kitzman et al., 2000, 2010; Olds et al., 1997, 1998, 2010; Olds, Kitzman, et al., 2004; Olds, Robinson, et al., 2004). The extensive research which has repeatedly shown positive outcomes has encouraged implementation in multiple states around the country.

Prevention Model Tier

The NFP is considered a secondary or tier 2 intervention since it provides services to a group of mothers who are at risk for having poor child outcomes due to poverty and not being experienced parents. The program is implemented for an extensive period of time with families but parents need only meet income requirements in order to qualify.

Parents as Teachers

Distinguishing Features

Parents as Teachers (PAT) can be distinguished from other parent training programs by the incorporation of multiple components including monthly in-home visits and parent group meetings, connecting parents to local resources, and yearly developmental screenings. Another defining feature is that the program is typically implemented as part of an agency's services to the community and not as a stand-alone curriculum. The program was developed in the 1970s in Missouri and was first implemented in 1981 to encourage family involvement in order to improve children's school readiness and school success. The program's goals have expanded to now also include (1) increasing parent knowledge of early childhood development and improving parenting practices, (2) providing early detection of developmental delay or health issues, and (3) preventing child abuse and neglect. The program is now implemented in all 50 states and in several countries.

Theoretical Grounding

PAT arose from the research literature which indicates that some children enter kindergarten already significantly behind their peers in terms of school readiness. By improving parenting practices early in the child's life, the program also focuses on improving parent–child attachment, a central aspect of John Bowlby's attachment theory. In addition, meetings with families teach skills via modeling and coaching, a connection associated with Bandura's self-efficacy theory.

Focus

The focus of PAT is to promote school readiness by working with parents from birth through age 5. The program has been implemented with primarily low-income families and with special populations including children with special needs, homeless families, teen parents, and incarcerated parents.

Time Requirements

The overall program is meant to work with families for 5 or more years, although this can vary depending upon the ages of children an agency works with (i.e., can be implemented by a preschool and only work with families for 2–3 years). The number of in-home visits and group meetings per month can also vary (weekly-monthly).

Child Participation

Children are only formally included in the developmental screeners which occur once a year. However, the individual meetings between parents and leaders can involve working on particular parenting issues with the child in the home.

Progress Monitoring Tools

The PAT website has printable Program Evaluation Handbook which provides many tools necessary for a local agency to examine the effectiveness and impact of the PAT services. In addition, the Outcomes Measurement Tool Kit provides information on a variety of measures that may be used by an agency to examine child and parent outcomes in multiple domains, depending upon the goals of the agency.

Training Requirements/Cost

Training is required for the different programs and services provided. However, this can vary by location, and practitioners are encouraged to contact the agency they are interested in working for to determine next steps for training. The trainings offered on the Born to Learn program cost between $520 and $700 depending upon location and also require the purchase of a guide ($295). Some supplementary trainings cost less due to the reduced content or narrowed focus. To find out about trainings, visit the website at www.parentsasteachers.org and click on the PAT University link.

Materials

For implementation of the program, parent educators are required to have the guides for the particular program they are using. In addition, agencies wishing to implement the PAT program need to have office space for parent educators including secure storage for family files and toys for home visits, as well as a meeting space for families and a play area for children. The PAT website has many materials available for practitioners including finding a local agency that is using PAT and reading suggestions grouped by various topics of interest to those serving children and families birth to age 5. Also available on the website are free tips and information for parents to assist their child's development in early academic domains (www.parentsasteachers.org and click the Parents portal and *Parenting Tips* link).

Empirical Support

Research on the outcomes of the PAT program has been extensive. Over 24 studies have been conducted to evaluate different aspects of the program. Regarding changes in parents, after receiving the PAT program, parents are more knowledgeable about child development, have better parenting skills, engage in more early learning activities, and are more involved in their child's schooling (McGilly, 2000; Pfannenstiel & Seltzer, 1989; Zigler, Pfannenstiel, & Seitz, 2008). Children of parents who participated in PAT were healthier and had higher early academic skills than children whose parents were not exposed to PAT (Drotar & Hurwitz, 2005; Wagner & Spiker, 2001; Zigler et al., 2008). A limitation to this research literature is that no randomized controlled trials have been used to compare outcomes of the PAT program to other established interventions or to a control group. Therefore, PAT is considered a *Possibly Efficacious* treatment.

Prevention Model Tier

The PAT program is a secondary or tier 2 prevention program. The program is designed to provide services to families at risk for poor outcomes and requires more time and resources than a primary prevention program.

Parent/Child Programs: Tertiary Prevention

A review of tertiary prevention programs revealed four programs: *Helping the Noncompliant Child Parent Training Program, Lovaas Applied Behavior Analysis, Parent–child Interaction Therapy,* and *Trauma-Focused Cognitive-Behavioral Therapy.*

Helping the Noncompliant Child Parent Training Program

Distinguishing Features

Helping the Noncompliant Child (HNC) can be distinguished from other programs by the very scripted session layout and the less stringent training requirements and lower cost. The therapy is divided into two phases: (1) teaching parents *differential attention* skills such as attending to positive behavior and providing rewards for desired behaviors, and (2) teaching parents' skills ensuring child compliance with requests. Several programs have arose from the original parent training therapy, including ones designed for groups of parents and a text for parents to use as a self-study. However, the primary program is still set up as a therapist working with each individual family (McMahon & Forehand, 2003).

Theoretical Grounding

HNC is grounded in theories which emphasize that challenging behaviors are shaped and maintained through patterns of family interactions that are maladaptive and serve to reinforce coercive behaviors (Patterson, 1975). The program was developed out of the Hanf Model of Parent Training (Hanf, 1969, 1970). This model focuses on teaching parents the skills of attending, rewarding, ignoring, providing clear instructions, and using time out appropriately (McMahon & Forehand, 2003). The training program also utilizes teaching strategies found within social learning theory (Sampers et al., 2001).

Focus

HNC is focused on addressing noncompliant behavior by improving parenting skills through modeling and role-play. The program is set to work with families of children ages 3–8 years old. In particular, the program intends to (1) establish positive and prosocial interactions between parents and their child, (2) improve parent skills in attending to positive behaviors, providing clear instructions, and providing consistent consequences for poor behavior, and (3) increasing child prosocial behaviors and decreasing conduct problems (McMahon & Forehand, 2003). The manual describes how to adapt the program for specific populations including children with ADHD, children who have been abused or neglected, and children with developmental disabilities or medical concerns (Wells, 2003).

Time Requirements

The length of time required to complete the program varies since completion depends on caregivers' ability to perform specific skills. In general, the families will require between 5 and 14 sessions that last 75–90 minutes each. Sessions should be scheduled twice per week to be the most effective. The sessions follow a very specific format (outlined in the manual) along with appropriate steps to teach each skill.

Child Participation

Children participate in sessions with their parents. The therapy room has a specific play area where the child will be most of the session, with parents practicing skills with their child while the therapist is present. The child is also informed about the parents' new skills throughout the program.

Progress Monitoring Tools

The primary text for this therapy contains all tools necessary to conduct sessions. At the beginning of each session, the therapist records the use of various skills taught during therapy on the Behavioral Coding System (BCS) for 5 minutes while the parent and child play. In addition, materials to conduct the initial interview, monitor parent progress, and gather gains in knowledge are included in the appendices of the text.

Training Requirements/Cost

Therapists are required to purchase the manual (*Helping the Noncompliant Child: Family-based Treatment for Oppositional Behavior*) and read it. It is available through multiple bookstores and costs approximately $60. The ISBN is 1-57230-612-2. In addition, a video tape that demonstrates intervention procedures and component parenting skills is available to assist with training. This video tape costs approximately $30 and is available from Rex Forehand at Child Focus, 17 Harbor Ridge Rd., South Burlington, VT 05403. There is also a leader's guide/manual for a 6 week parent class which can be obtained by contacting Nicholas Long at the Department of Pediatrics, UAMS/ACH, 800 Marshall Street, Little Rock, AR 72202.

Materials

Trainings can be completed in the home or in a clinic setting. The room should allow for a "play area" with toys that promote joint play and a second area with chairs for adults to sit and a chair placed further away for Time Out. The "play area" should not be near the door. Ideally, the session room would have a one-way mirror and the parent could have a "bug" in their ear for the therapist to guide them remotely, but this is not necessary. A supplemental book for parents that is a self-guided read and teaches similar skills is *Parenting the Strong-Willed Child: The*

Clinically Proven Five-Week Program for Parents of Two- to Six-Year-Olds. This text costs around $11 and can be found at most bookstores with the ISBN 978-0071383011.

Empirical Support

A long line of research supports the effectiveness of this program to increase compliance, decrease other problem behaviors, and improve parenting skills (McMahon & Forehand, 2003). When compared to other therapies (systems family therapy and STEP program), parents in the HNC groups had higher levels of positive and contingent attention and provided clearer instructions. Also, children in the HNC condition exhibited more compliance to adult requests and less disruptive behavior (Baum, Reyna McGlone, & Ollendick, 1986; Wells & Egan, 1988). While by and large the research supports the effectiveness of the program, there are some limitations to the research including the use of small samples that are predominately middle- or lower-middle class and of European American descent. However, HNC meets criteria for a *Well-Established* intervention program.

Prevention Model Tier

HNC is a tertiary or tier 3 prevention strategy when used with an individual family as this requires a large time commitment from the therapist. Although children do not require a formal diagnosis prior to treatment, to necessitate this level of care from a therapist, noncompliant behaviors must be a severe problem that has not been improved by previous interventions.

Lovaas Applied Behavior Analysis (Lovaas ABA)

Distinguishing Features

The Lovaas ABA model is a program designed for children with diagnoses that fall on the autism spectrum and can be implemented in two manners: clinic-based and consultation-based. Clinics are located in California, Indiana, New Jersey, and Pennsylvania. If a family is not located near a clinic, the family can enroll in the consultation-based track where a consultant will travel to a family to provide training and set up program goals. For the rest of this section, the consultation-based approach will be discussed. The Lovaas ABA program is unique in that parents assemble a team for their child of 3–5 individuals who in total will deliver approximately 35–40 hours of intervention per week. The intervention focuses on using shaping through task analysis-breaking down complex skills, teaching these smaller skills to the child, and shaping the skills into the complex behavior desired. Children must meet specific criteria in order to be assigned a consultant to train the child's team. To find out if a family qualifies, visit the program's website (www.lovaas.com) and click on *Enrollment*.

Theoretical Grounding

As can be expected, the Lovaas ABA method relies extensively on behavioral methods to teach children skills. The program does not necessarily focus on the specific ASD diagnosis, but instead focuses on the specific developmental delays a child is experiencing.

Focus

The focus of the Lovaas ABA model is to improve a child's areas of developmental delay that results from having a diagnosis on the ASD spectrum. The program accepts children as young as 18 months up through 8 years old, depending upon their developmental level. On occasion, children who are older than 8 years may be considered for intervention.

Time Requirements

The Lovaas ABA model requires extensive time of the child, with 30 or more hours being devoted to one-on-one intervention each week. The program can be carried out for multiple years with a child, depending upon their level of need and rate of progress in the intervention.

Child Participation

Children participate in all therapy sessions with either their parents or with another therapist. The therapy sessions often take place in multiple settings to have children use new skills and increase generalization of skills to the new settings.

Progress Monitoring Tools

The consultant that comes to the home relies on norm-referenced tests, parent interviews, and other ongoing assessments to track a child's progress. However, these assessments will most likely vary depending upon the child's areas of need.

Training/Requirements/Cost

Training costs are not listed on the program website.

Materials

The manual for the original program is entitled *Teaching Developmentally Disabled Children: The ME Book* and it is currently out of print. However, copies can be purchased from independent sellers through Amazon.com at a range of costs ($32.00–$75.00). To search for the book, use the ISBN number 978-0936104782. A newer version (*Teaching Individuals with Developmental Delays: Basic Intervention Techniques;* ISBN-978-0890798898) is also available and can be purchased through the Lovaas Institute's website at www.lovaas.com. The cost is $86.65. In addition to the manual, multiple other materials will be needed but these will vary depending upon the child one is working with and their particular needs.

Empirical Support

The Lovaas ABA method has 40 years of research to support aspects of the program. It meets criteria for a *Well-Established* intervention program. However, only two research studies will be reviewed as these were determined to meet rigorous research standards. The first study was conducted by Smith, Groen, and Wynn (2000). This study compared the Lovaas ABA method that carried out 30 or more hours per week for 2–3 years (15 parents) to an intense parent training condition where parents were taught the same approaches to use with their child in 5 hours a week for 3–9 months (13 parents). Results showed that at follow-up, children in the Lovaas ABA condition outperformed children in the parent training group on measures of intelligence, language, and academics, but not on adaptive functioning or behavior problems.

The second study (Sallows & Graupner, 2005) also compared a clinical Lovaas ABA condition to a parent condition with 13 children in the Lovaas condition and 10 children in the parent-directed condition. However, this time the parent-directed condition was modeled after the consultation approach currently used (parent leads a team of professionals who intervene with the child with minimal supervision). Interventions were carried out for 4 years and results showed that both conditions had positive outcomes for children in terms of increases in IQ scores, adaptive behavior, receptive language, and socialization. While these findings are promising, they do not represent replications by an independent research team and should be interpreted with caution.

Prevention Model Tier

The intense amount of time required to implement the Lovaas ABA model places this model into the third tier of prevention. Children typically have a diagnosis at the time they qualify for receiving a consultant.

Parent–Child Interaction Therapy

Distinguishing Features

Parent–Child Interaction Therapy (PCIT) can be distinguished from other parenting programs by the direct coaching parents receive and the performance-based termination. Parents receive direct coaching from the therapist during play with their child within the session. Also, therapy length can vary because therapists and parents agree on ending only when the parent is competent and confident enough to use the techniques taught on their own. The therapy is divided into two phases that address: (1) the parent–child attachment style, and (2) the skills of the parent in using authoritative parenting practices.

Theoretical Grounding

PCIT has developed out of Baumrind's (1967, 1991) developmental theory, which links child outcomes with various parenting styles (a more thorough review appears in Chap. 2 of this manual). A primary focus of PCIT is to assist parents with practicing authoritative parenting, a parenting style that results in positive outcomes for children. A second theoretical base for PCIT is attachment theory, with a focus on developing secure attachments between children and their parents. Finally, the techniques taught to parents within PCIT to manage behavior are drawn from social learning theory. By providing reinforcement for desired behaviors and removing reinforcement for aggressive or noncompliant behaviors in a consistent way, children's behavior will improve.

Focus

The focus of PCIT is on improving the parent–child attachment relationship and to improve the behavior management skills of the parent. Children are typically within the ages of 3–6 years old, although the program has been used with both younger and older children who exhibit disruptive behavior problems. Many of the children who benefit from this program have diagnoses of Oppositional-Defiant Disorder (ODD) or Conduct Disorder (CD) with comorbid Attention-Deficit/Hyperactivity Disorder (ADHD). PCIT has also been documented for use in cases where parents have been reported to state agencies for physical abuse.

Time Requirements

Sessions are planned to be approximately 1 hour long. A key component is that when teaching time out procedures for the first time during session, the session must be long enough so that the child eventually complies with the command. Also, the length of treatment can vary from 8 sessions to 20+ sessions depending on the severity of the behaviors and the parent's confidence with using the new skills and techniques. However, on average, completion takes about 15 sessions.

Child Participation

Children participate in sessions with their parent and the therapist.

Progress Monitoring Tools

Therapists keep track of how many times the parent uses the different skills taught within PCIT during the initial 5 minutes of the therapy session when the child and parent play together. This is coded on the Dyadic Parent–child Interaction Coding System (DPICS). Additionally, the Eyberg Child Behavior Inventory (ECBI)-Intensity scale is often completed prior to each session. This can yield criteria for completion, as termination is *not* recommended unless a raw score below 114 is obtained. Many of these tools are available from the website http://pcit.phhp.ufl. edu/ along with training information.

Training Requirements/Cost

Clinicians must have master's degree or higher in a mental health field and must be licensed in their field or receive supervision from a licensed individual trained in PCIT. Clinicians who meet requirements then complete a 40 hour face-to-face contact with a PCIT trainer. This most often occurs in a week-long workshop that costs $3,000. In addition to this, within 2–6 months of the initial training, an advanced live training occurs with real cases. This includes a minimum of two completed PCIT cases and maintaining regular contact with a PCIT trainer (via telephone, live observation, or tape review). Finally, skills must be reviewed by a PCIT trainer via videotapes, live observation, or online methods. This is the minimal level of training; clinicians can opt to attend further training and become a "Master Trainer" which allows them to provide training to other clinicians outside of the agency where they work.

Materials

Ideally, the sessions will take place in a room with a one-way mirror and the parent will have a device in their ear so the therapist can communicate with them. However, if this set up is not available, the therapist can sit in the corner of the room and coach the parent in a soft voice. Required materials include a chair and a room that can be used for the time out procedure along with toys and other activities for the parent and child to play together. Finally, the materials provided during the formal training include the PCIT manual to guide treatment.

Empirical Support

PCIT has a large research base indicating its effectiveness. Three rigorous trials have resulted in PCIT being named as a *Well Established* treatment for children ages 3–6 years old with disruptive behavior disorders (Bagner & Eyberg, 2007; Nixon, Sweeny, Erickson, & Touyz, 2003; Schuhmann, Foote, Eyberg, Boggs, & Algina, 1998). However, most of the participants within the study have been of European American descent (Brinkmeyer & Eyberg, 2003). More recent research has come out regarding the use with diverse groups and found a higher drop-out rate for African-American families, but treatment gains for completers were equivalent to or higher than other populations (Fernandez, Butler, & Eyberg, 2009).

A final area of research has been the use of PCIT with families with abusive behavior. Chaffin et al. (2004) found that parents who underwent PCIT were significantly less likely to have an additional report of abuse filed up to 3 years after ending PCIT sessions.

Prevention Model Tier

PCIT is considered a tier 3 prevention program. While a diagnosis of ODD, CD, or ADHD is not required, the children this intervention is typically used with do have these diagnoses. PCIT is very individualized and intensive. It is primarily conducted in individual sessions, requiring a large amount of time from the therapist.

Trauma-Focused Cognitive Behavior Therapy

Distinguishing Features

Trauma-Focused Cognitive Behavior Therapy (TF-CBT) is a program developed to assist young children and their families who have been through some type of traumatic event. TF-CBT works with both the child and the parent(s) in primarily separate sessions to process the trauma and create what is known as a "trauma narrative." The trauma narrative describes the trauma in detail to create a realistic representation of the event. Practitioners should note that this is one of the only evidence-based programs for young children who have experienced some type of abuse or trauma. In addition to this program, a cognitive-behavioral therapy for traumatic grief (TG-CBT) is available for older children (ages 6–17; Cohen, Mannarino, & Deblinger, 2006).

Theoretical Grounding

Several theories are evident in examining TF-CBT's programming. The program has both cognitive and behavioral components to assist children and their families in coping with the trauma. In addition, an ecological approach is taken that incorporates the entire family into the therapy process.

Focus

TF-CBT can be used with children ages 3–17 years old who are experiencing Post-Traumatic Stress Disorder (PTSD) or have subclinical levels of PTSD but are evidencing other difficulties in readjusting (e.g., behavioral problems, depression) after experiencing trauma or abuse. The program focuses on reducing the symptoms associated with PTSD such as reexperiencing events or remaining in a heightened arousal state. The program also seeks to increase the use of healthy coping mechanisms to handle stressors.

Time Requirements

TF-CBT is set up to be completed with the child in 12–18 sessions, with mostly separate sessions being attended by the parent. Sessions can last from 30 to 60 minutes depending upon the child's age and ability to participate with the therapist.

Child Participation

Children participate in their own separate sessions with the therapist to create the trauma narrative and process the trauma. In the parent sessions, parents are prepared to listen to the narrative and taught strategies similar to the child to reinforce use of these skills at home.

Progress Monitoring Tools

While no specific progress monitoring tools are detailed in the manual, studies of TF-CBT often track the effectiveness of therapy through use measures assessing PTSD, anxiety, and depression that are available to practitioners and specific to child ages.

Training Requirements/Cost

Training for TF-CBT is available online for free through the National Child Traumatic Stress Network and several other agencies at http://tfcbt.musc.edu/.

Practitioners who have a Master's degree or higher within a mental health discipline can register for the online training and are allowed to use TF-CBT after completing training and reading the manual.

Materials

In addition to the online training, therapists should purchase and read through the TF-CBT manual, *Treating Trauma and Traumatic Grief in Children and Adolescents,* which is available for purchase at most online bookstores for approximately $40.00. The ISBN number is 978-1-59385-308-2. In addition to the manual, practitioners should provide multiple art supplies to allow children options for creating their trauma narrative.

Empirical Support

TF-CBT has been investigated in multiple clinical trials, all with positive results. This has helped it meet criteria for a *Well-Established* therapy. The program has been honed through research to have the most impact through a combination of parent and child meetings, and to be conducted in as few as 12 sessions (Cohen et al., 2006). Children as young as 3 who have completed TF-CBT with their parents have been shown to exhibit reduced symptoms of PTSD, depression, behavior problems, and shame (Cohen, Deblinger, Mannarino, & Steer, 2004; Cohen & Mannarino, 1996, 1997; Deblinger, Lippman, & Steer, 1996). Parents who have completed TF-CBT report improvement in parental depression, distress related to the abuse, the use of positive parenting practices, and support of the child (Cohen et al., 2004; Cohen, Mannarino, & Knudsen, 2005).

Prevention Model Tier

Since TF-CBT is individualized and commonly conducted only with children and families who meet diagnostic criteria for PTSD, it is considered a tertiary level of intervention. The intervention works very intensely with family members to address trauma and/or grief.

Multi-tier Programs

There was one program that was best characterized as a multi-tier program, meaning that the goals of the intervention fit with multiple levels of prevention. This program is the Triple P program.

Triple P-Positive Parenting Program

Distinguishing Features

The Positive Parenting Program (Triple P) can be distinguished from other parenting programs by the comprehensive model put in place to deliver services to families with varying levels of need. The program's activities with families are divided among five levels which increase in intensity to meet the needs of families. Triple P's multiple formats can be implemented in different settings including the home, workplace, and clinics. The use of telephone consultation in several of the service delivery methods distinguishes Triple P from other parent training programs, allowing practitioners to reach families that live in rural areas or regions far from providers. It provides services for children from infancy to adolescence. The program was developed by Dr. Matthew R. Sanders at the University of Queensland, Australia, but the success of the program has resulted in adoption in multiple countries including the United States, Canada, and Germany.

Theoretical Grounding

Triple P draws from several theories to inform the multiple levels of service delivery. A primary method of changing behavior, Triple P draws from social learning theory and incorporates methods consistent with this theory to teach parents positive parenting strategies. An additional theory that Triple P is based on is the ecological model, and Triple P emphasizes that in order to impact problems, multiple domains where the problem occurs must be targeted. The program also pulls from research on family behavioral therapy which provides strategies to increase positive child behavior and decreasing the likelihood of problem behavior occurring. Triple P is also informed by research on development, including which factors are related to the development of challenging behaviors and psychopathology in children (Sanders, Cann, & Markie-Dadds, 2003).

Focus

The focus of Triple P is to provide services which promote the development of families that are independent and healthy. The program accomplishes this through promoting five parenting skills: (1) ensuring a safe and engaging environment, (2) creating a positive learning environment, (3) using assertive discipline, (4) having realistic expectations, and (5) ensuring parents take time to care for themselves (Sanders et al, 2003). In addition, families that are experiencing distress receive focused services on their respective needs (e.g., anger management, mental health concerns, marital discord).

Time Requirements

Time requirements to complete the intervention depend upon the level of intensity the intervention is delivered at. However, most sessions where a practitioner meets with parent(s) last from 1 to 2 hours. Within the program there are no more than 12 sessions with a family or groups of parents.

Child Participation

Depending upon which program within Triple P is used, children may or may not participate. In general, the programs within the higher levels of Triple-P (Levels 4 & 5) incorporate involvement of the child during the home visit or have parents practice newly learned skills with their children.

Progress Monitoring Tools

No measures are listed as progress monitoring tools on the program's website.

Training Requirements/Cost

To become a Triple P provider, practitioners must have a postsecondary degree in the fields of Health, Education, or Social Services and also attend Triple P training. The training is offered in two different formats: for individual practitioners and for organizations. For practitioners, Triple P training is held in Columbia, SC once a year and further information on dates and costs are available on the program's website (www.triplep-america.com). The cost for training varies between $1,450 and $1,905 and includes Triple P resources for the particular level a practitioner is trained on. Prior to registering, practitioners should check to make sure they meet prerequisites for their training, as some training sessions are sequenced.

If organizations want to adopt the Triple P system, training is available for all levels above the universal level (Levels 2–5) for up to 20 practitioners at one time. To find out more information about training in Triple P, email contact.us@triplep. net to request a quote. Included in the pricing for organizations is training, accreditation, training materials, practitioner manuals, and access to the web-based Triple P Provider Network with further information and resources.

Materials

Initial materials are included with the training. Additional materials are available by requesting a Practitioner Order Form from contact.us@triplep.net.

Empirical Support

Triple P has gathered empirical support for over 30 years of the program's implementation. Over 20 studies have documented a variety of positive outcomes (e.g., decreased problematic behavior, increased parent competence) for use with young children and preschool populations, helping this program acquire the status as *Possibly Efficacious.* Multiple studies have documented effectiveness with older populations. Therefore, a thorough review of the empirical support of Triple P is beyond the scope of this text. However, several consistent findings will be reported. The media campaign that composes the first level of services was investigated with 56 families (with 28 families watching the television series and 28 on a wait-list), and found that the families who watched the series reported lower levels of child behavior problems, higher levels of parenting competence, and rated this method of intervention delivery as very acceptable (Sanders, Montgomery, & Brechman-Toussaint, 2000). Regarding the delivery of parent training, in general, parents who completed any form of Triple P (self-directed, standard, workplace, or enhanced) reported reductions in: (1) child behavior problems, (2) parent mental health problems, and (3) parenting stress. Parents also reported higher levels of parent competence and more frequent use of positive parenting practices (Bor, Sanders, & Markie-Dadds, 2002; Connell, Sanders, & Markie-Dadds, 1997; Ireland, Sanders, & Markie-Dadds, 2003; Markie-Dadds & Sanders, 2006a, 2006b; Martin & Sanders, 2003; Roberts, Mazzucchelli, Studman, & Sanders, 2006; Sanders, Markie-Dadds, Tully, & Bor, 2000; Sanders et al., 2004; Turner & Sanders, 2006; Zubrick et al., 2005). Using Triple P has also been found effective in reducing marital/relationship discord in families (Dadds, Sanders, Behrens, & James, 1987; Ireland et al., 2003; Sanders et al., 2004), reducing feeding problems in young children (Turner, Sanders, & Wall, 1994), reaching and improving the lives of rural families (Connell et al., 1997; Dadds et al., 1987; Markie-Dadds & Sanders, 2006a, 2006b), and working with families where children are exhibiting behavior problems in combination with attention issues or developmental delays (Bor et al., 2002; Roberts et al., 2006).

Prevention Model Tier

Triple P has intervention services that cover all tiers of prevention. The program's Media Campaign (Level 1) provides information to all families, covering the primary prevention tier. The less intense parenting interventions (Levels 2, 3, and 4) consist of between 1 and 12 hours of instruction, provide information, and teach parents skills to handle moderately challenging behavior and to prevent further escalation of behavior problems. These elements would belong in the secondary level of prevention. Finally, the top level of services within Triple P (Level 5) provides intensive individualized services to families that have severe levels of child behavior problems coupled with other family issues. This level of service delivery falls into the tertiary level of prevention due to the severity of problems and the intervention's high demands for time placed on families and therapists.

Child/Classroom Programs

Commonalities Among Child/Classroom Programs

Before reviewing each of the child/classroom programs, it is helpful to recognize some of the commonalities among all of the programs which have a specific focus of improving outcomes for children. The child programs are delivered primarily through full-classroom instruction. However, a small subset of programs schedule meetings with small groups of children rather than the entire classroom. Much like the parent/child programs, most of the child/classroom programs employ a learning theory approach to teaching replacement skills. Other prominent theories utilized in these programs include Bandura's theory on the impact of modeling, Bronfenbrenner's ecological theory, and cognitive and developmental theories.

The programs that are reviewed have several common themes among them including (a) teaching children to identify emotions, (b) teaching prosocial skills related to self-control, (c) teaching children to problem solve, and (d) reducing problematic or aggressive behavior though behavior management. Additional areas programs focused on include promoting child resiliency and academic competencies.

The following programs are suitable for supporting children in prekindergarten or kindergarten settings according to EBP standards. While only four of these approaches have been documented for use with children under age 3, the description of these programs will help practitioners and parents determine which approaches might be most suitable for their child as they enter preschool age. As with the overview of parent/child approaches, information about training costs and materials is included to assist providers/funders in decision making. Table 5.3 below can serve as a broad overview of child/classroom programs reviewed in this chapter.

Child/Classroom Programs: Primary Prevention

Four child/classroom programs are at the primary level of prevention, meaning that the strategies are designed to assist all children. The programs within this section include: *Promoting Alternative Thinking Strategies, Second Step, Social Skills in Pictures, Stories, and Songs,* and *Tools of the Mind.*

Promoting Alternative Thinking Strategies (PATHS)

Distinguishing Features

The PATHS preschool program is a downward extension of a program that has proven effective in building social and emotional competence in older children. The

Table 5.3 Summary of child/classroom programs using PICO process

	Population	Intervention	Comparison	Outcome
Primary prevention program				
Promoting Alternative Thinking Strategies-Preschool Version	4–6 years	Classroom-wide affective education program	Possibly efficacious	Improved parent and teacher ratings of social and emotional competencies
Second Step	4–6 years old	Classroom-wide violence prevention program	Possibly efficacious	Improved ratings for social skills and disruptive behavior
Social Skills in Pictures, Stories, and Songs Program	3–5 years old	Classroom-wide adaptive skill building program	Possibly efficacious	Increased demonstration of social skills
Tools of the Mind	4–6 years old	Classroom-wide self-regulation and independence	Possibly efficacious	Improved ratings for behavior and self-regulation
Secondary prevention programs				
Al's Pals	3–8 years	Classroom-wide/small group resiliency and reduction of violence	Possibly efficacious	Reduced ratings for disruptive behavior and increased social skills
Devereux Early Childhood Assessment Program	2–6 years	Classroom-wide and parent training to develop child strengths	Possibly efficacious	Improvement in ratings for protective factors
I Can Problem Solve/ Interpersonal Problem Solving	4–5 years	Classroom-wide/small group affective and problem solving	Possibly efficacious	Lower ratings for problem behavior and increased problem solving
Incredible Years Dina Dinosaur Training	4–8 years	Classroom-wide/small group to promote self-control and compliance	Possibly efficacious	Improved ratings on child behavior measures when used with Incredible Years parent training program
Tertiary prevention programs				
Early Start Denver Model	12–60 months, with ASD	Intensive intervention including interventionists and parents	Possibly efficacious	Reduction in autism symptoms
First Steps to Success	4–5 years old	Screening with classroom and parent training	Possibly efficacious	Improved ratings on child behavior measures
Learning Experiences and Alternative Programs for Preschoolers and their Parents	12–72 months, with ASD	Individual and classroom-wide peer and adult-mediated strategies	Possibly efficacious	Reduction in autism symptoms, improvement in IQ and language

program can easily be integrated into the preschool curriculum. The authors note that PATHS extends previous work on social-emotional curricula by "including instruction in multiple skill domains that is delivered in a developmentally appropriate sequence" (p. 70; Domitrovich, Cortes, & Greenberg, 2007). The program includes activities throughout the curriculum to teach specific skills such as emotion labeling, complimenting, coping skills, communication skills, and problem solving.

Theoretical Grounding

The PATHS curriculum is grounded in Affective-Behavioral-Cognitive Dynamic model of development (Greenberg, Kusché, & Speltz, 1991) which explains the link of how affect, behavior, and cognitive understanding integrate to develop social and emotional competence. An additional theory that has influenced the program is Bronfenbrenner's ecological theory, with a primary focus in PATHS being the creation of environments that promote the use and generalization of new skills to other areas.

Focus

The primary goals of PATHS are to: (1) develop awareness and skills to communicate one's own emotions and the emotions of others, (2) teach self-control skills, (3) promote prosocial skills and positive self-concept, (4) build problem-solving abilities, and (5) create a positive classroom environment with structure that supports social and emotional learning.

Time Requirements

The PATHS program represents a year-round curriculum to be implemented in schools. The manual has 44 lesson plans that are divided into nine units to be covered over the course of a school year.

Parent Participation

No specific parent participation activities/strategies were mentioned on the website or in the seminal article on the preschool curriculum (Domitrovich et al., 2007).

Progress Monitoring Tools

The website (http://www.channing-bete.com/prevention-programs/paths/paths.html) provides a basic progress monitoring tool that allows teachers to rate changes in a child based on 31 different behaviors at the beginning and end of the school year (before and after the intervention). Also included for free are measures assessing the integrity and quality of lesson delivery and teacher satisfaction with PATHS. In addition, other measures can be included to assess specific behaviors or track a specific child's progress while receiving the PATHS curriculum.

Training

Training is conducted by certified, experienced trainers in a workshop format. For information on PATHS Preschool training costs, dates, and locations, select training workshops from the website.

Materials

The cost to implement the program is $479 per classroom. This price includes the teacher's manual, two curriculum manuals, storybooks for children, posters to display around the room, flashcards, and numerous other components related to the program.

Empirical Support

The PATHS preschool program has extensive research behind the elementary-age model and well-conducted research on the preschool model. In a randomized controlled trial of 246 children enrolled in Head Start classrooms, children who were in the PATHS Preschool program scored significantly higher than other children on measures of emotional and social competence. These differences were also observed by parents and teachers. Parents of children within the PATHS classrooms rated their children as more socially competent compared to peers and teachers rated children as more socially competent and less withdrawn than children who did not receive the PATHS curriculum (Domitrovich et al., 2007). This study along with the research support for the PATHS model has prompted the Substance Abuse and Mental Health Services Administration (SAMHSA) to add PATHS to the National Registry of Evidence-Based Programs and Practices. However, PATHS still requires additional replication research. Therefore, it is considered a *Possibly Efficacious* program.

Prevention Model Tier

The PATHS curriculum is considered a tier 1 prevention strategy as the program is delivered to all children within a classroom and the primary goals of the program are to promote social competence and thereby reduce problematic behaviors. The program can be incorporated into other curricula, increasing ease of use. Despite the long period of time the intervention is delivered (one school year), only 44 lessons are to be delivered, resulting in the time and resources needed to implement remaining relatively low.

Second Step

Distinguishing Features

Second Step is a curriculum that has different levels designed to be delivered to children from preschool through middle school. This section will focus on the Preschool/Kindergarten level. The program is under the ownership of the Committee for Children and has extensive research over the past few years to support its effectiveness.

Theoretical Grounding

Second Step is grounded in learning theory with regard to how skills are conveyed to students. Children are taught to observe and model prosocial behaviors and receive feedback and reinforcement for practicing new skills.

Focus

Second Step was developed as a violence prevention program. However, the primary focus is the reduction of problematic behavior by teaching children skills in empathy, emotion management, and problem solving. The level for preschool/kindergarten is designed for children ages 4–6 years old.

Time Requirements

Second Step for preschool has 25 lessons that are delivered twice a week for approximately 30 minutes. The program is spread across several weeks of the school year.

Parent Participation

Parents are informed of lesson content and are invited to watch a lesson through letters that are sent home. The letters also contain specific activities and strategies parents can use to encourage these skills at home and reminders to reinforce children for using new skills. In addition to these letters, a family guide is available in

English and Spanish and directs parents through six sessions consisting of videos and discussions. Take home handouts are included.

Progress Monitoring Tools

A number of assessment tools are available to progress monitor students and evaluate classroom implementation. These tools are included in the kit.

Training

Staff training is highly recommended prior to implementing Second Step. Training typically consists of 2 full-day workshops costing $525 per person. This cost includes a Trainer's Manual, staff training DVD's, and a training CD-ROM, but does not include the Second Step Kit. Information regarding trainings can be found at the Second Step website (www.cfchildren.org).

Materials

The cost of a preschool/kindergarten Second Step kit is $289.00. The kit includes all the lesson cards, teacher's guide, administrator's guide, three classroom posters, two puppets, a CD of songs, and a DVD for families to provide an overview. In addition, a supplementary pack is available for providing the lessons in Spanish for $69.00. All materials can be ordered through the Committee for Children's website (www.cfchildren.org).

Empirical Support

Two studies have examined Second Step preschool/kindergarten (McMahon, Washburn, Felix, Yakin, & Childrey, 2000; Moore & Beland, 1992). However, only one study could be obtained (McMahon et al., 2000). Fifty-six preschool children (from primarily African-American and Latino backgrounds) participated in Second Step. The results of a pre-test/post-test comparison revealed that the children had increases in their knowledge of social skills and decreases in observed aggressive and disruptive behavior. Further research is needed to support the program and examine the effectiveness of the parent component, thus it is considered *Possibly Efficacious*.

Prevention Model Tier

Second Step is a primary prevention program because it is delivered to all children and focuses on promoting behaviors inconsistent with problem behaviors.

Social Skills in Pictures, Stories, and Songs Program

Distinguishing Features

The Social Skills in Pictures, Stories and Songs Program (SSPSSP) can be distinguished from others by the use of a self-determination approach as a method of increasing adaptive skills and decreasing problem behavior. The program originated under the name "Living with a Purpose." SSPSSP is intended to be implemented as a component of a preschool curriculum. The premise behind SSPSSP is that providing children with the ability to have input into decisions that affect their lives will lead them to be more resilient. The skills are taught through stories and coloring books and children are given the opportunity to act out skills and receive feedback.

Theoretical Grounding

The SSPSSP is grounded in learning theory with regard to how skills are presented to children. Children are taught to observe and model particular behaviors and receive feedback and reinforcement for practicing new skills.

Focus

SSPSSP focuses on four adaptive skill areas: (1) following directions, (2) sharing, (3) managing one's behavior, and (4) problem solving. It can be delivered in English and Spanish and is intended for children between the ages of 3 and 5 years old.

Time Requirements

The SSPSSP program is carried out over 12 weeks by having two 3-hour sessions each week within the classroom.

Parent Participation

No specific parent involvement strategies are included.

Progress Monitoring Tools

No tools are included in the materials and none were mentioned on the website which the program could be ordered through (www.researchpress.com).

Training

In the research that has been conducted, teachers observed a Master Teacher for at least 3 months prior to implementation and received a manual. Training can be provided to teachers by request, and costs will vary depending upon the needs of the teachers (L. Serna, personal communication, August 10, 2010). To schedule training, contact Loretta Serna, Ph.D., at rett@unm.edu or 505-277-0119.

Materials

The materials are available for purchase through www.researchpress.com. The cost for the complete kit is approximately $150.00 and an additional ten sets of coloring books are available for $50.00.

Empirical Support

Three trials of the SSPSSP have been conducted comparing classrooms that received the intervention and classrooms that did not (control). The results of the first trial were quite impressive, with teacher ratings of the SSPSSP classrooms improving after the intervention (Serna, Nielsen, Lambros, & Forness, 2000). In addition, children who exhibited significant emotional and behavioral problems prior to the SSPSSP either improved or were no worse after the intervention. However, similar children in the control classrooms either became worse or demonstrated symptoms of new emotional and/or behavioral disorders (Serna et al., 2000). A limitation to this trial was that the teachers implementing the intervention were highly trained.

The second trial had typical teachers implement the SSPSSP curriculum within Head Start classrooms. Differences between the SSPSSP and control groups were much smaller, indicating lesser effects of the intervention and possible issues related to measurement error (Serna, Nielsen, Mattern, & Forness, 2003). In the third trial, the methods from the second study were repeated, but structured observations focusing on measuring the specific skills taught in the program were also included. This third replication had similar findings to the second regarding small differences between groups on ratings of emotional and behavioral symptoms, but did find that children who received the SSPSSP intervention increased their use of the SSPSSP skills from 20–40 % to 90–100 % (Serna, Forness, & Mattern, 2002).

Several limitations should be noted within the replication studies and be considered prior to implementing this program, including: (1) lack of independent replications, (2) the program has only been studied with children attending Head Start, and (3) in all studies, raters and observers were aware of whether or not the children were receiving the intervention. Due to these limitations, SSPSSP meets criteria as a *Possibly Efficacious* treatment.

Prevention Model Tier

SSPSSP is a primary prevention program because it is delivered to all children and focuses on promoting behaviors that will lead to resilient children.

Tools of the Mind

Distinguishing Features

Tools of the Mind (TM) is a preschool classroom curriculum that focuses on preparing children for elementary school by developing self-regulation skills. The program makes use of play throughout the classroom day to develop specific skills in language, rule-learning and ability to follow rules, interaction with peers and adults, and to develop specific skills associated with self-regulation. The core of TM is 40 strategies that promote the development of self-regulation, and the use of these strategies composes 80 % of a child's day (Diamond, Barnett, Thomas, & Munro, 2007). The program began as a collaboration between Drs. Elena Bodrova and Deborah Leong and has been implemented in Colorado, Florida, Maine, Massachusetts, New Jersey, New Mexico, North Carolina, Oregon, Pennsylvania, Tennessee, Texas, and Washington. TM has also been adapted for use within a kindergarten classroom and to accommodate the special needs of children with disabilities or developmental delays so that these children can remain integrated in the regular classroom.

Theoretical Grounding

The TM program is grounded in Vygotskian theory of child development and relies heavily on the concepts of scaffolding and zone of proximal development (Barnett et al., 2008). Teachers use specific strategies within the classroom to scaffold a child's learning. This involves providing a lot of assistance as a skill is initially learned and gradually removing that assistance as the child becomes able to perform the skill independently. The zone of proximal development refers to the gap that occurs between what a child can accomplish independently and what level of performance can be achieved with assistance from another person.

Focus

The focus of TM is primarily on the development of self-regulation through play. By developing self-regulation skills, children within the classroom should be able to learn more easily because they can direct their own attention and ignore distractions, reflect on their thinking, remember better, and engage in more prosocial behaviors with peers and adults (Leong, 2009). The program also emphasizes critical early learning skills in the areas of literacy, numeracy, science, and writing.

Time Requirements

Tools of the Mind is used throughout a school year and can be implemented in half-day and full-day preschool settings.

Parent Participation

No specific activities are mentioned involving parents within the program description or research literature.

Progress Monitoring Tools

No specific tools are mentioned to monitor child progress. However, one of the program developers indicates that the progress of children and the class as a whole is monitored, daily, weekly, and monthly (Leong, 2009). The program also has fidelity checklists available for program coaches or administrators to use to monitor how well the TM curriculum is being implemented.

Training

Training in TM is conducted as part of a regimented 2-year implementation plan. To begin implementation, a team must be created within the district that is composed of at least teachers, assistant teachers/paraprofessionals who will be implementing TM, administrators of the preschools, and a site coordinator or coach for the district. During the first year, the curriculum is divided into four phases and coaches and other team members attend four workshops that correspond with these phases. Also during this year, the preschools receive four on-site visits by TM trainers to ensure that the newly acquired skills are being implemented correctly. The first year of training covers: development of self-regulation through play, management of the classroom, planning and developing rich play themes for use within the classroom, and activities to teach literacy, math, and science skills. Special education staff can also receive training on the Response to Intervention (RtI) model. The second year of training for preschool settings focuses on: individualization of activities, accommodating children with special needs, and assessment of child learning. The content and number of workshops is negotiated with TM staff to meet the ongoing needs of the district.

Costs of training are based on a per classroom price for a district and can be determined by contacting the person below (Leong) responsible for the region in which the program will be implemented. Leong (2009) indicated that the average cost of first year training during 2008 was $2,000–$3,000 per classroom and the cost of second year training was typically around half of the first year. This training cost does not include training for special education staff, which is contracted on a per person basis. For more information on training, contact Training@ToolsoftheMind.org.

Materials

The TM program utilizes materials that are commonly used within a preschool classroom as well as some tools that are TM-specific. Typical TM classrooms include at least one teacher and an assistant teacher or paraprofessional within each classroom, but this may vary depending on the class size. The staff at the TM primary office can assist districts that wish to implement TM by suggesting modifications, adaptations, and additions to current materials the district possesses. The staff can be contacted through the program's website (www.toolsofthemind.org) to determine needed materials and relative costs of implementation.

Empirical Support

The TM program is supported by 15 years of research in kindergartens and preschools; however, randomized trials have only been published more recently. A randomized trial of 21 classrooms compared the TM curriculum with a Balanced Literacy curriculum that covered similar academic content, but did not emphasize self-regulation. Children who were in TM classrooms performed better on self-regulation tasks than children in the other classroom condition (Diamond et al., 2007). While these results are strong, they do not provide information about differences in academic achievement, which is an important outcome.

A second randomized trial took place in New Jersey and again evaluated the differences between TM and a curriculum that covered the same academic content but reflected the school district's traditional instructional delivery. A total of 7 classrooms implemented the TM curriculum and 11 classrooms offered the "traditional" instruction. Results indicated that the TM curriculum was significantly better at improving classroom behavior and children's self-regulation skills. However, early academic outcomes did not show significant differences between conditions (Barnett et al., 2008). With this research, TM meets criteria for a *Possibly Efficacious* program.

Prevention Model Tier

The TM program should be considered a tier 1 level of prevention since it is delivered to all children within the classroom. The program focuses on preventing behavior problems in all children by developing aspects of self-regulation, skills documented to improve multiple outcomes for children.

Primary or Secondary Prevention Programs

Four programs were found that had the ability to address children's needs at the primary and secondary levels depending upon how the program is delivered. The programs that can be delivered in a classroom-wide or small group format are *Al's*

Pals, the *Devereux Early Childhood Assessment Program, I Can Problem Solve,* and the *Incredible Years Dina Dinosaur Training Program.*

Al's Pals

Distinguishing Features

Al's Pals consists of two different curricula for children ages 3–8. *Al's Pals: Kids Making Healthy Choices* (AP-KMHC) is a curriculum designed to be implemented in a classroom setting throughout the school year. *Al's Caring Pals: A Social Skills Toolkit for Home Child Care Providers* (ACP-SST) is a program which provides training and materials to help children develop social skills and healthy decision making.

Theoretical Grounding

Al's Pals curricula focus on the promotion of resiliency in children. A lesson is taught to children, which is reinforced by modeling and role play.

Focus

The intent of Al's Pals is to increase resiliency and reduce future substance abuse and violence by emphasizing prevention in children ages 4–5 years old. The primary goals of the program are to increase protective factors within a child's life by increasing their social-emotional competence and decrease the known risk factors of early and persistent antisocial and/or aggressive behavior (Lynch, Geller, & Schmidt, 2004).

Time Requirements

The AP-KMHC program is composed of 43 lessons lasting approximately 20 min long. The lessons are designed to be given over 23 consecutive weeks.

Parent Participation

No specific parent involvement strategies are included. However, letters are sent home to parents explaining what their children are learning within the AP-KMHC curriculum. Also, a separate program known as *Here, Now and Down the Road* is available for parents to participate in. This is not required to be delivered at sites delivering the child program(s).

Progress Monitoring Tools

No specific progress monitoring tools are included with the program.

Training

Training is available through workshops practitioners can attend, on-site trainings arranged with the company, and a web-based training for both programs. If training occurs in a face-to-face format, it is typically conducted in a 2-day workshop. The online training is conducted in seven 2-hour segments that are spread out over a few weeks. To find out costs of different training methods for a particular practitioner or group, contact the company by visiting the website: www.wingspanworks.com/contact_us.

Materials

The various materials for the Al's Pals program are available after completing training. Depending upon the particular program desired and the needs of the setting in which it will be implemented, costs vary.

Empirical Support

The AP-KMHC program has been evaluated during implementation for four school years in a row between 1993 and 1997. All evaluations of the AP-KMHC program have included control classrooms. The evaluations over the years showed that AP-KMHC program decreased ratings of behavior severity on the Child Behavior Rating Scale (Dubas, Lynch, Galano, Geller, & Hunt, 1998). Many sites continued to implement the program in all classrooms and provide data to the owners of the program for the 1997–2000 school years. The information from these centers indicates that the children increased their prosocial behaviors, social interaction, and positive coping skills (Lynch et al., 2004). These findings support the effectiveness of the program when implementation is not strictly controlled or conducted by highly trained teachers. The results of these studies indicate that AP-KMHC does meet criteria for a *Possibly Efficacious* treatment. As of publication of this guide, the ACP-SST program does not have any published research regarding its effectiveness.

Prevention Model Tier

Both programs could be considered as fitting into the primary level of prevention. However, since the *Al's Caring Pals* program is used more often with a smaller group of children, it could also be considered a secondary level of prevention since it could be used to give more extended instruction to children who may be struggling with behavior and/or emotional concerns.

Devereux Early Childhood Assessment (DECA) Program

Distinguishing Features

The DECA Program can be distinguished from other early childhood programs due to the primary emphasis on problem solving to identify and strengthen protective factors. A central component of this program is the use of the DECA Assessment within a five-step problem-solving process. The first two steps entail gathering information and administering the DECA to assist with problem identification. The third step is to summarize and interpret results as a method of problem analysis. The fourth and fifth steps are to develop and implement a plan to address the identified problem and then to evaluate child progress through multiple methods, respectively. The DECA program has been adapted for infant and toddler ages (DECA-I/T), children (DECA), and children who are school-age (DESSA). However, research has primarily focused on the DECA. Therefore, the DECA program will be reviewed in detail.

Theoretical Grounding

The DECA Program is grounded in research focused on resilience, or the achievement of positive outcomes despite adverse conditions (Wyman et al., 1999). By developing child strengths known to lead to positive outcomes, children are better equipped to handle stressors that occur within their life.

Focus

The DECA is designed to be used with children ages 2–6 years old. Within the intervention plans, there is an explicit focus on developing the protective factors of initiative, attachment, and self-control as a method of reducing behavior concerns.

Time Requirements

Most research on the program has used the strategies as part of a year-long preschool curriculum. No information was found on the website regarding implementing the strategies for less time. Additionally, no information was found on how long or how often DECA-specific strategies were used with children.

Parent Participation

The DECA program has a parent information source on promoting resilience in children entitled *For Now and Forever.* This text provides parents with simple strategies that can be implemented at home to extend skills being taught within the preschool setting.

Progress Monitoring Tools

Several tools are available to monitor child progress throughout the use of the DECA program. These are included with the purchase of the kit, although more are available for purchase through Kaplan. The tools include an observation journal, parent and teacher rating forms, and pre- and post-test tables. The DECA is also available in a web-based format which allows for data entry of information into a computer system. For more information on the forms and web-based DECA, visit www.kaplanco.com.

Training

DECA trainings are scheduled several times a year in multiple locations around the country. Those who are allowed to attend the training and learn to use the DECA include mental health professionals and early childhood professionals with graduate level training in assessment. If a practitioner does not have this level of training, he or she can attend a training and pass a competency assessment to be allowed to use the DECA. To find out information about training options, such as locations, scheduling, costs, and types of training, contact the Devereux Early Childhood Initiative at 866-872-4687.

Materials

The program kit is ordered through Kaplan (www.kaplanco.com). The entire kit, which includes user manuals, parent and teacher guides, record forms, and a strategy guide tied to the outcomes of the DECA assessment, costs approximately $200. Additional parts are available for purchase including parent guides and record forms in Spanish ($25–$40) and a set of children's books which focus on teaching positive skills ($160).

Empirical Support

A total of three unpublished studies were found that examined the effectiveness of the DECA assessment and program strategies in combination. The first two studies involved the piloting of the program in its entirety (Devereux Early Childhood Initiative, 2000; Lebuffe & Likins, 2001). The first 2 years of the pilot study included 545 preschool children split into a DECA-exposed group and a control group. The DECA-exposed group utilized the DECA assessment and program strategies throughout the school year. Some problems were noted with the reliability of teacher reports for use as measures of growth over the year. However, parent reports in both studies and teacher reports in the second year indicated that children within the DECA-group had increased levels of protective factors and decreases in behavior concerns.

A final study (LeBuffe, 2002) consisted of a DECA-exposed group and a control group which completed pre-test and post-test measures on protective factors and behavior concerns. Both measures were completed by parents and teachers. Regarding behavior outcomes, the control group showed worsening behavior ratings by both parents and teachers over the course of the school year. In contrast, children in the DECA-group had maintenance of behavior scores (i.e., no change from pre-test to post-test). In the protective factors ratings both groups showed improvements, with the DECA-group showing more improvement than the control group, although the differences between groups were not statistically significant.

All these data should be interpreted with caution because (1) differences between groups have not been statistically significant (2) the research has not gone through a peer review process, and (3) no independent replication studies have been conducted with other research teams. For these reasons, the DECA program is rated as *Possibly Efficacious*.

Prevention Model Tier

The DECA program can be used as a primary or secondary level of prevention, depending on if it is used with all children in a preschool classroom or just some who are identified as at-risk. Depending upon the number of strategies needed to assist a child and the resources required to implement these strategies, the program could be classified as a secondary level of prevention.

I Can Problem Solve/Interpersonal Cognitive Problem Solving (ICPS)

Distinguishing Features

The ICPS program has been developed through more than 30 years of research on interpersonal problem solving. The program is delivered to an entire classroom and is divided into two phases. The first phase focuses on teaching children the language necessary for problem solving, ensuring that they understand the meaning of the words. Examples include the words *different, not,* or *because.* The second phase of the program teaches children how to recognize specific emotions and the specific steps from problem solving. The overall focus of the program is to teach children *how to think* instead of instructing them *what to do.* This is accomplished through the use of games, stories, puppets, and role-playing.

Theoretical Grounding

The ICPS program heavily relies on cognitive components to accomplish problem solving. In addition, the use of role-playing and modeling incorporate Bandura's theory that children will repeat behaviors they see others engaging in.

Focus

The purpose of the program is to assist children in identifying emotions and learning and using problem-solving skills in order to reduce interpersonal conflict. The program is used primarily with older preschool children (ages 4–5) and has been implemented primarily with children who come from low-income, urban environments.

Time Requirements

The program is implemented over a 12-week period, with 20 min lessons being delivered every day of the week (59 lessons total). In addition to the scripted sessions, teachers are encouraged to use the problem-solving language when problems appear for children throughout the day to generalize skills beyond the planned intervention practice sessions.

Parent Participation

Parents can participate through a parallel program entitled *Raising a Thinking Child Workbook*. The workbook teaches parents to use dialogues at home that are similar to the ones used in school and include children in problem solving at home. The workbook is available in English and Spanish at www.researchpress.com and costs $23.95.

Progress Monitoring Tools

No tools are mentioned for progress monitoring on the Research Press website.

Training

Depending upon location, on-site training may be arranged. Costs, length of training, and availability vary. To arrange for staff training, contact Dr. Myrna Shure at 215-762-7205 or at mshure@drexel.edu.

Materials

The only material needed is the program manual, which is available through Research Press at www.researchpress.com. The manual costs $41.95. All materials can be replicated from the manual.

Empirical Support

A number of research studies have been conducted on the ICPS program dating back to 1976. The ICPS program was originally investigated in preschool and kindergarten classrooms, with studies indicating that children who complete ICPS generate more solutions to problems and have improved behavior ratings by teachers (Shure & Spivack, 1979, 1980, 1982). The ICPS program was also independently replicated with a preschool sample in rural Michigan (Feis & Simons, 1985). The results of this 3 year study found that children in the ICPS group were able to generate more potential solutions to problems and able to generate a wider array of solutions. In addition, the ICPS group also had lower ratings of problem behavior compared to controls (Feis & Simons, 1985). The replication of the ICPS program in a less-structured environment with a different population and still achieving similar outcomes lends support to the program's effectiveness. However, studies have documented that the program does not significantly reduce aggressive behavior in young children (Feis & Simons, 1985; Rickel & Burgio, 1982). The ICPS program is therefore rated as *Possibly Efficacious.*

Prevention Model Tier

This program falls into the primary prevention tier, since it is used with entire classrooms. However, the program can be used with small groups of children who are struggling with demonstrating correct behavior in class. In the latter situation, the program would be considered a secondary level of prevention.

Incredible Years Dina Dinosaur

Distinguishing Features

The Incredible Years Dina Dinosaur Training Program (DDTP) can be distinguished from other interventions since it has been adapted for use with small groups or as a prevention program within a classroom setting. DDTP is meant to be used with children between the ages of 4–8, with lessons adapted for different ages (Webster-Stratton & Reid, 2003).

Theoretical Grounding

DDTP is grounded in research focusing on specific behaviors which predict later aggressive and noncompliant behavior. By remediating these behaviors early on, the program seeks to reduce the likelihood of developing conduct disorder (Webster-Stratton & Reid, 2003). The program takes a social learning approach to teaching skills which integrates Albert Bandura's self-efficacy theory to promote the use of new prosocial skills within children. The self-efficacy influence is evident in the emphasis on modeling and practice within each session.

Focus

The DDTP focuses on reducing noncompliant and other problem behavior by teaching social skills and play skills, promoting the use of self-control strategies, providing knowledge on labeling feelings, practicing perspective taking, and boosting academic success and confidence. As a result of participating in the program, children typically have increases in self-esteem and self-confidence and reductions in defiance, aggressive behavior, bullying, stealing, lying, and other behaviors associated with noncompliance.

Time Requirements

The small group format is designed to be carried out in 22 sessions held once a week. Each group meeting lasts about 2 hours and can be held in conjunction with the parent training meetings. The classroom curriculum is delivered throughout the school year, 2–3 times each week in a 20–30 minute block.

Parent Participation

Parents participate in the Incredible Years training program, often at the same time as their children. Often the parents will attend a BASIC training which covers initial principles and then continue training with a secondary set of parent trainings that focuses on advanced skills or promoting school success, depending upon the child's age. Although the parent and child curricula are aligned, no joint meetings between the groups are planned.

Progress Monitoring Tools

A number of progress monitoring tools are available for free on the program's website (www.incredibleyears.com). The child outcomes are measured through two forms of assessments: games and classroom observations. The two "game" assessments focus on labeling feelings from the perspective of others and assessing what a child might do in a social situation by asking them to describe their behaviors. Both these assessments have separate prompts for boys and girls and inquire about situations that are relevant to children. The classroom observation tools codes child behavior, classroom environment, and teacher behavior to determine changes that may have resulted from the program.

Training

The training requirements for the child program are similar to the other Incredible Years programs. However, depending on the professional role of the group leader, the training set-up may differ. If a classroom teacher plans to implement the child curriculum in the classroom, training is typically completed in four 8-hour days which may be completed in 1 week or be spread out over a few weeks. The certification process for other professionals follows a similar pattern to the training for the parent program, with workshops lasting approximately 3 days and costing around $400. Information for all trainings can be found on the Incredible Years website at www.incredibleyears.com. Like other Incredible Years programs, additional training is required to become a certified group leader or a certified mentor, which allows providers to provide training with the title or to train other providers, respectively.

Materials

The DDTP complete kit for small groups is $1,150 and the classroom costs a little bit more ($1,250) due to the inclusion of five lesson plan manuals.

Empirical Support

Two randomized control trials have been conducted which include an evaluation of the DDTP (Webster-Stratton & Hammond, 1997; Webster-Stratton, Reid, & Hammond, 2001a). The initial study examined the impact of various combinations of the Incredible Years Programs compared to a control group. The three groups that received intervention were given either extended parent intervention, parent intervention and child intervention, or only the child intervention (DDTP). Results of the initial trial showed that all treatment conditions resulted in positive outcomes for families (reduced problem behavior and increased use of prosocial skills), but the conditions that included DDTP also resulted in improvements in child problem solving and conflict management skills (Webster-Stratton & Reid, 2003). These changes were maintained when families were followed up with 1 year later, but the strongest impact was evidenced by the group which received both the parent and child training. For this reason, these programs are recommended to be used together.

The second trial investigated whether teacher training resulted in further improvement in outcomes since the initial study revealed that children had *increases* in problem behavior at school at the 1-year follow-up (Webster-Stratton & Reid, 1999). The results of this study suggested that adding teacher training to the child and parent trainings results in reduction of problem behaviors at school and home (Webster-Stratton et al., 2001b). Thus, DDTP is rated as *Possibly Efficacious.*

Prevention Model Tier

If the program is used as a classroom curriculum, the intervention can be considered as a tier 1, or primary prevention strategy. This is because all children are receiving the intervention and it is designed to promote prosocial skills in order to prevent problem behavior. If the program is used with a small group of children (ideally 6 or less; Webster-Stratton & Reid, 2003), it should be considered as a secondary prevention approach (tier 2). This is because the small group will require more resources and the curriculum is a more focused intervention for these children who are already deemed at risk for developing problem behavior.

Classroom Programs: Tertiary Prevention

Three programs require extensive time and effort from practitioners. The use of these programs should be reserved for children with very challenging behaviors. These programs are *Early Start Denver Model, First Step to Success,* and *Learning Experiences and Alternative Programs for Preschoolers and Their Parents.*

Early Start Denver Model

Distinguishing Features

The Early Start Denver Model (ESDM) was created by Sally Rogers & Geraldine Dawson and represents an intensive early childhood intervention for children diagnosed with autism spectrum disorders (ASD) not arising from a chromosomal abnormality. The program combines multiple interventions which have been used with children who have been diagnosed with ASD, including techniques which are associated with Applied Behavior Analysis (ABA), and those that are non-ABA. In addition, this model is designed to be implemented with a team of early childhood professionals that can address multiple areas of child development.

Theoretical Grounding

ESDM utilizes an eclectic approach that incorporates multiple theories to understand development and theories specific to the impact ASD has on child skills. Since the ESDM is a combination of Pivotal Response Training and the Denver Model, it also draws upon theories of social learning and cognitive development (Piaget), respectively.

Focus

The focus of ESDM is children between the ages of 12 and 60 months, although some reports vary as to exact age ranges. The ESDM is designed as a comprehensive developmental behavioral intervention that improves developmental outcomes in multiple domains (e.g., communication, socialization, cognition, and adaptive behavior).

Time Requirements

The program is very time-intensive, with one-on-one therapy occurring for 20 hours per week (two 120 minutes sessions each weekday) with the child. The program is implemented in this manner for 2 years. In addition, other therapies (e.g., occupational, speech) are carried out in conjunction with, but at a separate time from, ESDM training sessions.

Parent Participation

Parents participate in a separate parent training component which meets for 12 sessions (90 minutes each session) and is then followed by four 90 minutes follow-up visits. The parent training consists of teaching parents to implement techniques from the ESDM (Vismara & Rogers, 2008).

Progress Monitoring Tools

Progress is to be monitored with the Early Start Denver Model Curriculum Checklist which is available in sets of 15 for $48.00 from multiple bookstores. Within the practitioner's manual there are also example forms that can be used to track child progress on specific objectives.

Training

Implementation of ESDM requires extensive training. Prerequisites for training include: (1) having a postbaccalaureate degree in a field related to education, (2) working regularly with children 1–4 years old who have autism, and (3) having the resources necessary to submit training materials to the training center for fidelity checks. The website provides a step-by-step process for practitioners (www.ucdmc. ucdavis.edu/mindinstitute/research/esdm/). However, a brief outline is provided here: (1) purchase and read the ESDM manual (ISBN: 978-1606236314) and curriculum checklists (ISBN: 978-1606236338)—each costs approximately $48.00, (2) attend the sequence of trainings (introductory, advanced, parent coaching, and trainer of trainer) which cost $375 per training, and (3) after each workshop, submit two rounds of products for certification purposes and to receive feedback. The training is sequenced so that practitioners must become certified for one workshop before registering and completing the next workshop in the sequence. All trainings are currently held in Sacramento, but on-site trainings can be arranged with the authors. To request an on-site training or gather more information, practitioners can call email megan.manternach@ucdmc.ucdavis.edu.

Materials

Besides the manual and checklists, multiple other materials are needed to implement sessions. Practitioners are directed to the manual and curriculum checklists for complete lists of required and suggested materials.

Empirical Support

One randomized control trial was found for ESDM (Dawson et al., 2010) and several other studies were noted by the program authors to be in press, but not yet available. In the Dawson et al. (2010) study, the authors reported a number of positive outcomes (i.e., changing diagnosis for Autism Spectrum Disorder to Pervasive Developmental Disorder—Not Otherwise Specified, increases in IQ) and a number of flaws within the study and the measures used for evaluation are not addressed. Due to these flaws, caution is recommended in interpreting the claims of the effectiveness of the program. In particular, outcomes of the second year of implementation were not significantly different from first year outcomes, indicating that the second year of extensive intervention may not yield large improvements. Thus, ESDM is rated as *Possibly Efficacious.*

Prevention Model Tier

Due to the extensive number of resources required to implement this program in a similar manner to the research that has been conducted, this program would fall into the third tier of prevention. For children to utilize these services, they require a diagnosis of ASD.

First Step to Success

Distinguishing Features

The First Step to Success (FSS) Program has programs available for preschool and kindergarten levels. FSS is composed of three unique modules. The first component involves universal screening to determine which children are at risk for not developing appropriate skills. In the second module, parents, teachers, and a consultant work together to develop contingencies for an identified child within the classroom so that the child may earn rewards at school for him/herself and his/her classmates as well as at home based on behavior. The final component of the program involves the consultant working with the parents to teach and have their child practice new skills to improve their behavior (Walker, Severson, Feil, Stiller, & Golly, 1998).

Theoretical Grounding

The FSS program is grounded in social learning theory. The program also heavily emphasizes a prevention perspective, theorizing that using early and intensive interventions for at-risk children will reduce behavior problems and negative long-term outcomes. Finally, the incorporation of parents into the modules supports the program's ecological perspective.

Focus

The FSS program for preschool is designed to be used with children who are between the ages of 4 and 5 years old. Children are identified as likely to develop severe problematic behaviors.

Time Requirements

The intervention is carried out throughout the year, but the formal intervention period in classrooms is around 30 classroom days (Powell & Dunlap, 2009). However, the intervention may be extended or altered depending on the child's response to separate components.

Parent Participation

Parents of a child who has been identified as at-risk for poor outcomes due to risk factors in their background and their problematic behavior participate in the program. During the time where the child is receiving the intervention in the classroom, parents are to reward children once they arrive home on days where the target behavior is achieved. In addition, parents participate in training sessions, one-on-one with the consultant, to develop and implement interventions to reduce or eliminate problematic behaviors at home.

Progress Monitoring Tools

No progress monitoring tools are provided. However, progress is documented based upon each child's individual needs and goals.

Training

For information on training, contact the program's author, Hill Walker, Ph.D., at (541) 346-2583 or by email at hwalker@oregon.uoregon.edu.

Materials

The kit for preschool costs $166.49 and is available from http://store.cambium learning.com. The kit includes an implementation guide, Home-Based Coach guide, Parent handbook, and an overview video. In addition, a resupply kit is needed for each new group of children the program is implemented with. The resupply kit is available from the same website and costs $53.95 and includes materials for one additional implementation. However, the most essential component of the program is a well-trained consultant who can effectively implement the FSS program.

Empirical Support

All of the research on FSS focuses on children who are in elementary schools (kindergarten through second grade). No research was found regarding the effectiveness of the preschool application of the program. However, studies on the kindergarten program have shown that children who complete the FSS program fall within the normal or typical range on measures of aggression, time engaged in class activities, and adaptive and maladaptive behavior rating scales (Golly, Sprague, Walker, Beard, & Gorham, 2000; Lien-Thorne & Kamps, 2005; Russell Carter & Horner, 2007). Also, the changes observed in children have been maintained for 1–2 years after the intervention was implemented (Epstein & Walker, 2002). Since the research is limited to Kindergarten, no criteria is met for determining the evidence base for the preschool curriculum. Thus, FSS is rated as *Possibly Efficacious*.

Prevention Model Tier

The FSS program is considered a tertiary level prevention program since it works intensely with one child who is displaying problematic behaviors. The coordination of multiple interventions in multiple settings (i.e., home and school) makes this program a more complicated intervention than others placed at lower tiers.

Learning Experiences and Alternative Programs for Preschoolers and Their Parents (LEAP)

Distinguishing Features

LEAP is a preschool curriculum that focuses on inclusion of children with autism in a typical classroom. The classroom is set up to have 10 typically developing children and 3–4 children with autism. LEAP uses typically developing peers within the classroom to increase social interactions. Teachers review the specific goals of the children with autism on a weekly basis and measure progress toward these goals. The curriculum used within the classroom is designed to meet the needs of children who fall developmentally between the ages of 12 and 72 months (Strain, 1987). Other professionals besides the classroom teachers are brought in on an as-needed basis, such as speech pathologists or occupational therapists. The program also includes a family component described below. This program should not be confused with Kennedy Krieger's LEAP program (Lifeskills and Education for Students with Autism and other Pervasive Behavioral Challenges), which provides intensive serves to children ages 5–21 in a noninclusive setting.

Theoretical Grounding

LEAP incorporates social learning theory and developmental theory (Strain, Kohler, & Goldstein, 1996) throughout all aspects of class-wide and individual intervention. Also included within the program is an emphasis on peer- and adult-mediated strategies within interventions to assist children with autism in developing new skills. To unify the diverse needs, the curriculum used within classrooms, *The Creative Curriculum* (Dodge & Colker, 1988), serves as a general guide to programming activities.

Focus

The goal of the program for the children with autism is to promote development and improve skills in social, emotional, language, adaptive behavior, cognitive, and physical domains. LEAP does this by exposing children with autism to preschool activities that typically developing children would engage in and by only adapting the curriculum when it is deemed necessary (Strain et al., 1996)

Time Requirements

Children attend the school setting year-round for 15 hours each week (3 hours/day). In addition, parent training is offered at multiple points during the year.

Parent Participation

Parent involvement is essential within the LEAP program (Strain et al., 1996). Parents can participate by completing activities within the classroom, or by attending a parent education program. Also parents of children who have moved out of LEAP may provide information or support to newly enrolled parents (Strain et al., 1996). In the parent training portion of the program, parents are taught skills and how these skills can be implemented in multiple settings (Strain, 1987). In later phases of the parent training, parents develop and implement interventions to assist their child as well as gather information on the interventions' effectiveness (Strain, 1987).

Progress Monitoring Tools

Most studies used progress monitoring tools specific to the behaviors of concern. These included observational tools and rating scales such as the *Childhood Autism Rating Scale* (CARS; Schopler, Reichler, & Renner, 1988).

Training

Teachers must have a master's level degree in an education or related field. No further information regarding training is available. To find out more about the curriculum, the LEAP Outreach Project can be contacted via the Teacher's Toolbox website or at 866-811-8665. To inquire about training opportunities, contact Ted Bovey, M.A., at ted.bovey@cudenver.edu or by phone at 303-315-4934.

Materials

A variety of materials are needed to implement this program since it is a full preschool curriculum. Children engage in a number of activities throughout the year and engage in play in multiple centers which must be filled with toys that prompt child-led play and specific social skills.

Empirical Support

The LEAP Program and its individual components have had numerous studies that support the effectiveness of the program. While a thorough review of the research is beyond this section, a few key findings are presented. After 2 years of being enrolled in a LEAP preschool, children with autism show reductions in autistic symptoms and increases in intellectual and language domains (Hoyson, Jamieson, & Strain, 1984; Strain & Cordisco, 1993). Typically developing children have no documented negative outcomes and several positive outcomes including better social skills and fewer disruptive behaviors (Strain, 1987). With regard to the family component, family members who have participated in the LEAP program are significantly less likely to show signs of stress and depression when compared to families not enrolled in the program (Strain, 1987). The evidence supporting the LEAP program has been consistent and for that reason it is considered to be a scientifically based best practice for working with young children diagnosed with autism (Simpson, 2005) and meets criteria as a *Possibly Efficacious* treatment.

Prevention Model Tier

Because the LEAP program requires children to have a diagnosis of autism for particular students to be included and a number of resources must be devoted to the classroom, this program falls into the tertiary level of prevention services. However, providers should note that a continuum of services are provided to children diagnosed with autism. Most interventions occur on a class-wide level, with some components of the program being implemented in a small group or individual basis.

Conclusions

Children's development can best be supported by attending to their relationships and the environments in which they live, including home, school, and community settings. Evidence-based programs are available to address multiple risk factors, enhance caregivers' skills, and improve children's prosocial skills which lead to more optimal outcomes for children and their families. EBPs are often organized within a prevention framework, which enable families, schools, and communities to provide the care and nurturing that children need by informing them about development and reserves the most intensive resources to address the needs of those most at risk.

The two primary formats for delivery of services include parent/child interventions and child/classroom curricula. In either case, the purpose of the intervention is to help children reach their full potential, so that they can be happy, healthy, and productive individuals. Depending upon the program, services may be provided in the home, school, or other community setting. Some intervention packages even allow for individual, self-paced instruction. The skills and competencies needed to improve development can be taught to children, parents, and other caregivers. In the case of children with diagnosed conditions such as autism spectrum disorders, interventions become more labor-intensive, require additional preparation on the part of the trainer, and as such, become more expensive to deliver. More research is needed to document interventions which are effective, responsive, culturally sensitive, and developmentally appropriate and can be used in evidence-based practice.

Assess Your Knowledge

1. What program is commonly conducted out of a medical clinic or pediatrician's office?

    a. Triple P
    b. Incredible Years
    c. Nurse-Family Partnership
    d. Reach Out and Read

2. Which program can only be carried out by a registered nurse?

    a. Helping Our Toddlers, Developing Our Children's Skills
    b. Nurse-Family Partnership
    c. Reach Out and Read
    d. Parent–Child Interaction Therapy

3. Which program is *NOT* considered a well-established treatment according to the Chambless and Hollon (1998) criteria?

    a. Parent–Child Interaction Therapy
    b. DECA Program
    c. Incredible Years
    d. Helping the Noncompliant Child

4. Which program requires no formal training beyond familiarizing oneself with the manual?

    a. Helping the Noncompliant Child
    b. Parents as Teachers
    c. Reach Out and Read
    d. Nurse-Family Partnership

5. Which of the following programs is *NOT* specifically designed for children diagnosed with Autism Spectrum Disorders?

    a. Lovass ABA
    b. First Step to Success
    c. Early Start Denver Model
    d. Learning Experiences and Alternative Programs for Preschoolers and Their Parents (LEAP)

6. Which of the following programs can *NOT* be used in a small group format?

    a. Lovaas ABA
    b. Dina Dinosaur
    c. I Can Problem Solve
    d. Al's Pals

7. Joanie was physically abused by one of her relatives for 6 months. The abuse has stopped, but she is experiencing nightmares and avoids entering the neighborhood where the abuse occurred. Which program might be best for her?

   a. Trauma-Focused Cognitive Behavior Therapy
   b. Early Start Denver Model
   c. First Step to Success
   d. Devereux Early Childhood Assessment Program

8. Representing the importance of developing this skill in early childhood, which of the following is a focus in the majority of early childhood interventions?

   a. Developing problem-solving skills
   b. Identification of emotions
   c. Self-control
   d. All of the above

9. Which intervention combines a parent/interventionist team to address one child's problem behavior?

   a. Dina Dinosaur
   b. I Can Problem Solve
   c. Early Start Denver Model
   d. Promoting Alternative Thinking Strategies

10. Which two programs focus specifically on increasing child resiliency in order to cope with future stressors?

   a. The Devereux Early Childhood Assessment Program & Tools of the Mind
   b. Tools of the Mind & Promoting Alternative Thinking Strategies
   c. Al's Pals & the Devereux Early Childhood Assessment Program
   d. Promoting Alternative Thinking Strategies & Al's Pals

Assess Your Knowledge Answers
1) d   2) b   3) b   4) a   5) b   6) a   7) a   8) d   9) c   10) c

Chapter 6
Behavioral Terms and Principles

Abstract Many evidence-based interventions for addressing challenging behavior in young children utilize behavioral strategies. This chapter outlines key behavioral principles (e.g., reinforcement, punishment, schedules of reinforcement and punishment, extinction, imitation, shaping) that can be used to prevent and intervene with problem behaviors in young children.

Keywords Reinforcement (positive and negative) • Schedules of reinforcement • Punishment • Extinction • Imitation/modeling • Shaping • Time out • Social stories

There are a number of interventions designed for parents and providers to help young children exhibiting challenging behaviors. Many are behaviorally based, with the goal of increasing desired behaviors and reducing maladaptive behaviors. Behavioral principles incorporated into each of these programs have been shown to be effective in decreasing challenging behaviors and increasing desired behaviors. A solid understanding of behavioral principles will help professionals understand behavior and decide which intervention strategies are likely to be the most effective in modifying behavior. In addition, learning the common terminology will facilitate communication between professionals and caregivers. This chapter will describe the basic principles of behavior, including how behaviors are learned and maintained. Specifically, this chapter will outline the following behavioral principles:

- Reinforcement (positive and negative)
- Punishment
- Schedules of reinforcement and punishment
- Extinction
- Imitation/Modeling
- Shaping

K.H. Armstrong et al., *Evidence-Based Interventions for Children with Challenging Behavior*, DOI 10.1007/978-1-4614-7807-2_6,
© Springer Science+Business Media New York 2014

Reinforcement

Reinforcement occurs when the consequences following a behavior increase the likelihood that the behavior will reoccur in the future. It is important to point out that reinforcement in the technical sense refers to anything that results in an increase in behavior. The reinforcement does not have to be something the adult believes will be reinforcing to the child. For example, a child may be reinforced for hitting their parent by the parent yelling at the child. Even though the parent intends their yelling to be a punishment, whether or not it is reinforcement is dependent on the effect it has on the child's behavior. If the child continues to hit after the parent has yelled at their child, the yelling is likely serving as reinforcement to the child.

Immediate reinforcement has the greatest effect on influencing a child's behavior. Research suggests that even a delay of 1 min before presenting the reinforcer may inadvertently reinforce another behavior (Malott & Suarez, 2004). This concept becomes very important to understand in instances when children have very brief occurrences of desired behavior, such as eye contact or communication. If reinforcement does not occur immediately a child may not understand what behavior is being reinforced.

Unconditioned reinforcers refer to those reinforcers which do not have to be learned and function similarly for all people. These reinforcers include food, water, warmth, and touch. Conditioned or learned reinforcers are those which become powerful through association with other reinforcers, and after the association is made, can function as a reinforcer. Learned reinforcers include tokens, money, points, etc., and can be used to shape desired behaviors. Reinforcers may also be classified as edible (snacks or bits of food), sensory (vibration or lights), tangible (trinkets or stickers), activity (play or special events), or social (attention; Cooper, Heron, & Heward, 2007). Attention is one of the key reinforcers for behavior in young children, and includes behaviors such as looking, smiling, patting, or praising. Reinforcers are as unique as people are. Therefore, it is useful to find out what children like before developing any intervention plan. Parents and caregivers can often tell you what their child likes the best, and in some cases, children can tell you. In the case of very young or nonverbal children, pictures can be used to help them choose reinforcers.

Parental attention (proximity, eye contact, words) can be a powerful reinforcer for young children, and can be used to strengthen many behaviors: the good, the bad, and the ugly. For example, if caregivers comfort a child when he has a tantrum, lay down with a child who repeatedly gets out of bed, or laugh when a child passes gas, their attention will reinforce the very behavior which the caregiver possibly does not want to see their child repeat. On the other hand, when caregivers praise a child for waiting her turn, compliment the child for sharing her toy, or notice when the child speaks in an inside voice, the attention will reinforce these behaviors which are more desirable, and increase the likelihood that the child will repeat the behavior in the future.

There are two types of reinforcement: positive reinforcement and negative reinforcement. *Both* lead to an increase of the behavior in the future. The "positive" refers to presenting or adding something following a behavior. An example of positive reinforcement is praising a child after she goes to the potty. Praise becomes a reinforcer for going the potty, and will increase the likelihood that the child will go to the potty in the future. Both positive and negative reinforcement are said to "strengthen the behavior," making the behavior more likely to occur in the future.

"Negative" refers to withdrawing or removing something aversive following a behavior, which reinforces the behavior. An example of negative reinforcement is turning off a vacuum to stop a child from screaming. Turning off the vacuum can be said to be negative reinforcement, because it may increase the child's screaming in the future to avoid aversive noises. Negative reinforcement provides the person with a sense of relief, making it more likely for the person to repeat the behavior under similar conditions in the future. Negative reinforcement is often confused with punishment, as both terms are associated with aversive conditions. However, negative reinforcement leads to an increase of future behavior (child's screaming stops mom's vacuuming, thereby teaching child that screaming stops the aversive noise), while punishment results in a decrease of behavior (mom spanks child to stop the child's screaming). Punishment will be discussed in more depth later in this chapter.

Negative reinforcement within parent–child interactions creates a response pattern that can lead to the development of oppositional and aggressive behavior. Patterson and his colleagues (1975, 1989) coined the term coercive process to describe such parent–child interactions in which attention is rarely provided for desired behavior, aversive exchanges increase, and discipline is inconsistent and becomes harsher over time. In the early stages of the coercive process, a parent may say to her child "no candy today" while in the grocery checkout line. The child whines, cries, and starts yelling, and mother feels everyone in the store looking at her and is embarrassed. Ultimately, the parent gives in, and allows the child to have the candy, avoiding any more embarrassment. In the end, reinforcement operates for both the child and parent. The child is reinforced for disruptive behavior by getting the candy, and the parent is relieved that everyone stops looking at her. When these interactions occur over time, the parent will become harsher towards the child, and the child will become even less compliant. A child may become quite adept at this pattern of behavior, and will interact like this with other adults such as teachers and coaches, as well as with peers.

Punishment

Punishment refers to any event that weakens a behavior, and reduces the likelihood that a behavior will occur in the future. Just as with reinforcement, punishment can be thought of as positive or negative, depending upon the change within the environment. An example of positive punishment is spanking a child following misbehavior. An example of negative punishment is time out following misbehavior,

Table 6.1 Relationship between reinforcement and punishment

Effect on behavior	Present a stimulus following the behavior	Withdraw a stimulus following a behavior
Strengthens behavior	Positive reinforcement	Negative reinforcement
	Reinforcement by adding a consequence	*Reinforcement by removing a consequence*
	Example: giving attention for sharing with another child	Example: turning off a loud appliance after a child screams
Weakens behavior	Positive punishment	Negative punishment
	Punishment by presenting a consequence	*Punishment by removing a consequence*
	Example: spanking a child is the consequence for stealing a toy	Example: aggression results in loss of attention

because a child is removed from the opportunity to receive attention. Similar to reinforcement, punishment is more effective in producing behavior change when it occurs immediately.

Like reinforcement, there are many types of punishment. What works best in suppressing the behavior depends to a great degree upon the individual's history, and the immediacy and intensity of the punisher. According to Cooper et al. (2007), when punishment is used, it should occur immediately and consistently after the problem behavior, and be supplemented by reinforcement of the desired behavior.

Punishers can include time out, loss of privileges, verbal reprimands, and anything else that follows a behavior and weakens it. What is important to remember about punishment is that sometimes punishment is effective in stopping an unwanted behavior. Used sparingly, saying "no" firmly to a young child may reduce unwanted behavior. However, punishment must be used selectively and carefully, in order to minimize undesired side effects. For example, caregivers who depend upon punishment (verbal reprimands, spanking, and time out) for discipline may find that they must become firmer and harsher to achieve the desired effects. In addition, punishment may stop a behavior, but does not teach the child the desired behavior. Therefore, whenever punishment is used as part of an intervention plan, it should *always* be paired with some strategy to encourage the desired behavior. Lastly, frequent use of punishment can create bad feelings between the caregiver and the child, and damage their relationship. Table 6.1 below displays the relationship between reinforcement and punishment.

Schedules of Reinforcement

Schedules of reinforcement (and punishment) refer to the timing of the event (reinforcer or punisher) following the behavior, and are important to consider when teaching children new skills and maintaining established behaviors. There are four basic schedules of reinforcement: Fixed interval, fixed ratio, variable ratio, and variable interval, as well as more complicated schedules which are beyond the scope of this text. Interval schedules occur when the fact that the reinforcement or punishment is based on time, while ratio schedules are based on the number of responses needed for reinforcement. Fixed schedules are consistent, while variable schedules are unpredictable. With these definitions in mind, a variety of different scheduling types can be constructed. Fixed interval schedules are when the time requirement for reinforcement remains constant. Variable interval means that the timing of the reinforcement is random. Fixed ratio refers to a set number of responses which must occur before reinforcement. Variable ratio indicates that reinforcement will occur after a random number of behaviors.

There are different effects upon behavior and learning, depending upon the schedule of reinforcement. Continuous reinforcement (or reinforcement provided for each behavior) is more effective when teaching new behaviors, while intermittent reinforcement helps to make behaviors more durable and long-lasting. Interval schedules tend to produce low to moderate rates of response (Cooper et al., 2007). Fixed interval schedules often result in a pattern of response that picks up as the reinforcement is anticipated, and then drops off following reinforcement (imagine how productive that last few minutes are when a child has been asked to clean up all toys in 5 min). Fixed and variable ratio schedules often produce high rates of responding. Variable ratio schedules tend to produce a more consistent response than fixed ratio. In other words, if you don't know how many times you need to do something (e.g., how many stickers a child needs to earn) before being reinforced, you may be more likely to continue to respond at a steady rate.

Time Out

Time out is a form of punishment, which is used to reduce problem behavior by removal of the opportunity to receive attention or access to positive reinforcers for a specific amount of time. Time out is an effective disciplinary method for children between the ages of 3–12 years old, however time out is not recommended for use with younger or older children (McMahon & Forehand, 2003). The programs *Helping the Noncompliant Child* (McMahon & Forehand, 2003) and *Parent Child Interaction Therapy* (Eyberg, Nelson, & Boggs, 2008) have both designed specific time out sequences that parents and early childhood professionals can follow. Below we have provided some guidelines to follow when implementing time out.

Setting Up Time Out

Step 1: Decide which behaviors will result in time out. A rule of thumb is to use time out only for the most serious behaviors, including aggression and repeated noncompliance.

Step 2: Decide where time out will take place. The ideal time out locations are *boring spots* where the child cannot damage items and there is nothing of interest. Good places often include a hallway or the dining room. Time out places should never be scary (i.e., closets, bathrooms, rooms without lights).

Step 3: Make sure parents understand that they are NOT to engage with their child in any way during time out. We recommend the use of a timer to eliminate parent reinforcement.

Step 4: Teach the child about time out: why he must go there, where it will be, what behavior is expected, how long time out will last, and what happens after time out is over. If other children are in the home, make sure they understand that when someone is in time out they should be ignored.

Using Time Out

Time out typically works well for noncompliance or aggression. The following procedures should be followed immediately after observing aggression or after a second prompt to comply with an adult request is not followed. Early childhood professionals can teach parents and other caregivers these steps, and they may also use them in their own practice. Several other specific versions of a timeout sequence can be seen from Zisser and Eyberg (2010), or McMahon and Forehand (2003).

1. The caregiver should escort the child to the time out area.
2. The caregiver should give the child a brief explanation for why the child is being placed in time out ("You are going to timeout because you hit your brother") and a clear instruction for what they are to do ("Please sit quietly on the mat until I tell you that you can get up").
3. The caregiver should avoid arguing or discussing anything further with the child here, and should turn their attention away from the child.
4. The caregiver should keep track of the time that the child is in time out and follow the rules that they have set with the child in advance (e.g., that the child must be quiet while in time out, how long they need to stay there).
5. Based on what the offense was that landed the child in time out, the caregiver should address the child at the end of the time out by referring back to the issue (e.g., "are you ready to clean up your toys?" "are you ready to tell your brother you are sorry?").
6. If the child agrees and subsequently follows through, the child can return to playing.
7. If the child does not stay in the time out area, the caregiver should return the child to the time out area, reset the timer, and give the child a clear command to stay in the time out area until they say they can get up. This is repeated until child successfully completes time out.

Options for Younger Children

Since time out is generally used with children 3 or older, a modified or softened version of time out can be used with children under age 3. This procedure is more commonly used for children under 3 years old who have acted aggressively (not as frequently with noncompliance). After observing an aggressive act, a parent should:

1. Remove the child from the person they were aggressive with (to another part of the room or to another room).
2. Remove attention from the child who was aggressive but remain with them.
3. Wait until the child has calmed down before talking to them.
4. If appropriate and the child has the verbal skills, the child can be reintroduced back to the area and apologize to the child who received the aggression.
5. Play then returns to normal with praise for appropriate behaviors.

This adapted form of time out keeps other children safe and does not have expectations that are above and beyond a toddler's limits of ability (sit in the chair, stay by yourself). It can also prevent the child from developing poor strategies socially since aggressive behavior is not allowed to "pay off" because the child is removed from playmates and toys.

Extinction

Extinction refers to a process by which behavior is reduced or eliminated, because it is no longer being reinforced. Extinction involves systematically ignoring unwanted behavior that is maintained by attention, which gradually eliminates the behavior. If parental attention is thought to be maintaining the problem behavior, the caregiver can consistently ignore the child when he is engaging in the behavior, and it will eventually go away. This is referred to as "planned ignoring."

Problem behavior often gets worse before it gets better, which is referred to as an "extinction burst," and in the case of attention, the child's behavior may actually escalate to gain the parent's attention. Thus, the early childhood professional must provide fair warning that despite their hard efforts to ignore challenging behavior, their child's behavior is likely to get more difficult at first, and they must not give in to these demands. Caregivers can be informed that more challenging behavior may be a sign that the intervention is working. Consistency is key in any intervention to modify or extinguish unwanted behavior through planned ignoring. As with other punishments, positive reinforcement for desired behaviors helps children learn what behaviors are acceptable and which are not.

A related concept that uses extinction is the concept of differential attention. Differential attention combines extinction with reinforcement to quickly change a child's behavior. To use differential attention, a caregiver ignores all unwanted behaviors and provides praise and attention for behaviors that are desired. An example would be when a child is playing in an inappropriate way (i.e., drawing and talking about poop being in the toilet), a parent using differential attention would ignore this behavior. As soon as the child begins to talk about or draw more appropriate objects (i.e., alligators in a lake) the parent would provide attention to the child, possibly saying, "What a great alligator! I love how you used so many colors to make him!"

One note for using extinction, planned ignoring, or differential attention is that these strategies should never be used with clearly aggressive behaviors. Aggressive behaviors should be addressed through redirection and sparing use of punishment.

Extinction: Differential Attention

Every time 5-year-old Lisa and her mother go to the grocery store, Lisa whines through the entire trip until her mother gives in and buys her candy. Lisa's mother cannot stand the whining and is embarrassed when other people look at her ill-behaved child. Lisa's mother decides to use differential attention to stop this behavior.

On the next visit, Lisa begins pleading for candy shortly after they enter the store. Lisa's mother ignores her behavior, and Lisa begins to whine louder and louder. Soon, Lisa is screaming and pulling things off the shelves as they go through the aisles. Lisa's mother calmly removes her child's hands for the shelf and guides her out of the store to their car. Lisa's mother was ready for the extinction burst, and she stays with her plan of ignoring Lisa's inappropriate behavior. She does not give in and buy Lisa candy.

Lisa's behavior is less disruptive the next time they go shopping, although she still whines, her mother continues to ignore her, and goes about shopping. Whenever Lisa does something positive, her mother praises her. After two more visits, Lisa has stopped whining, and is able to enjoy the shopping trip.

Imitation/Modeling

Imitation refers to the process of learning new behaviors through the observation of others. From the earliest stages of development, babies watch their caregivers and begin to imitate their behaviors. Just as with other behaviors, reinforcement strengthens the modeled behavior. Research has documented that modeling behaviors depends upon many variables, including how closely the child identifies with the model, how powerful the model appears to be, and whether the model is reinforced for the behavior (Bandura, 1977). Children with autism or other developmental disabilities may have difficulty naturally imitating others; however, they may be taught to do so, thus modeling can be used to teach new behaviors (Garfinkle & Schwartz, 2002).

Since caregivers are so influential to their children, they must be very careful not to model inappropriate behaviors, because their child is likely to behave in a similar fashion. For example, if a parent drops a cup, and then uses inappropriate language in front of a child, the child might also do the same. If the parent then says "Oh no!" and laughs, thereby reinforcing the behavior, the child is likely to repeat this behavior again. Also, modeling of behaviors does not stop with observing caregivers. Children will model behavior that they observe in other children, characters they see on television, and video characters.

Modeling and Imitation

Vincent is 5 years old and is watching his favorite TV show, Teenage Mutant Ninja Turtles. The show has four turtle characters that fight crime in the city through martial arts techniques. Later that week, Vincent is on the playground with a group of four boys. The boys decide that one child is their sworn villain and begin spin-kicking him and throwing "ninja stars" (sticks) at him. His friends cheer him as he spin kicks the villain.

This change in Vincent's behavior is best explained by imitation as he did not engage in these types of behaviors prior to watching the show. One event that strengthened the likelihood that these behaviors would be imitated is that the Teenage Mutant Ninja Turtles were often rewarded for their fighting actions. Secondly, Vincent's friends reinforce him for his actions.

Modeling can become a powerful teaching tool to develop children's social skills. Exposing young children to peers or siblings who are able to share, take turns, and use words to express themselves provides powerful examples of prosocial behavior. Modeling becomes even more influential if the model is reinforced for their good deeds, and if the child imitating this behavior is also reinforced. By clearly pointing out and reinforcing the peer's good choices, caregivers will discover that their child shortly demonstrates the same behavior, and should praise him or her.

Modeling and Imitation

Sean is 2 years old and is playing with his older sister, Alicia (age 5). Alicia is playing with one of her more interesting toys and sees her brother reach out for it. At that moment, Alicia gives the toy to Sean. Their father, having seen the entire interaction, praises Alicia saying, "Alicia! Thank you so much for sharing your toy with your brother!" He wishes to reinforce Alicia's good behavior and point out that this behavior is what he likes to see from both Alicia and Sean.

Later, Sean is playing with blocks with his sister. When his father comes around, he picks up a block and hands it to his sister saying, "Sharing!" Sean's father praises him for sharing with his sister.

Using Stories to Facilitate Imitation/Modeling in Novel Situations

Social stories are tools that can be used to teach children how to behave in situations that might be new to them, such as going to school, or for scenarios that they usually have difficulty with, such as going to the doctor's office. These stories can be particularly useful for children diagnosed with autism spectrum disorders (ASDs); however, they can be used effectively with any child. Social stories include both text and pictures and are written from the perspective of the child. The ratio of text and pictures is selected by the age and developmental level of the child. For example, younger children will need more pictures and less text than older children. Social stories typically include a mix of descriptive, perspective, and directive sentences. It has been recommended that a story should include 3–5 descriptive and perspective sentences for every directive (Gray et al., 1994).

After creating a social story, the story is shared with the child numerous times so that the child can learn the skills embedded within the story. The text essentially provides a model for the child to follow in a difficult situation. The text from a sample story appears in Fig. 6.1:

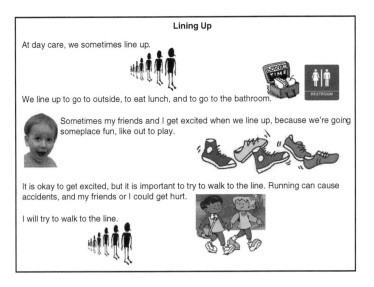

Fig. 6.1 Sample social story

Shaping

Shaping refers to a process of setting a behavioral goal, then breaking down the goal into smaller, more attainable steps, and combining both positive reinforcement and ignoring to achieve the goal. This strategy is often used by teachers to develop skills that a child has not yet mastered, and ensures that the child will be have success with each step in the right direction.

An example of shaping the behavior of using words for requests would be to first show the child a desired object, such as a cookie, prompt the child to say "cookie," offer praise for approximations of the word, and reinforce the child by giving him the cookie. As the child becomes more proficient in requesting with one word, the demands are gradually be increased, so that the child is expected to eventually say "I want cookie please." The key to shaping behavior is having knowledge of which skills the child already possesses, understanding which steps are needed to reach the desired goal, and gradually increasing behavioral expectations towards the goal.

Shaping is a very helpful tool that allows parents and caregivers to help children attain behavioral goals by reinforcing the "baby steps" towards mastery. It is unrealistic to expect that a child will master a complicated behavior without first mastering the foundational skills, so the skills needed to reach the desired goal are broken down into easier to manage approximations, and progress is reinforced. Shaping is a teaching technique that utilizes all of the principles of reinforcement to reach the desired behavior.

Conclusions

Documented through years of careful research, the application of behavioral principles has been shown to improve human behavior and developmental outcomes. Early intervention professionals must acquire a solid understanding of behavioral principles, how they influence behavior, and how to use these strategies successfully in order to improve the lives of the children and families they serve. The next chapter will go into more detail on how to apply behavioral principles in everyday practice.

Assess Your Knowledge

1. After a child kicks the dog, his parents laugh. The child now kicks the dog daily. For the child, this is an example of:

   a. Positive punishment
   b. Positive reinforcement
   c. Negative punishment
   d. Negative reinforcement

2. A preschool teacher reports that they have "punished Johnny" for hitting his peers by having him sit in the corner. Johnny's hitting behavior has actually increased since this "punishment" has been implemented. Is having Johnny sit in the corner an effective punishment?

   a. Yes
   b. No
   c. Not enough information to tell

3. In the past, if Ethan threw a tantrum when his mom was running errands, she would immediately go home. Ethan's mom has decided to try to eliminate this behavior by ignoring the tantrum and continuing to run errands. She notices that the first time she tries this method, Ethan's tantrum is worse than usual. What is the term to describe this?

   a. Extinction
   b. Punishment
   c. Extinction burst
   d. Reinforcement

4. A therapist wishes to teach a child how to verbally ask for a snack instead of crying, and thinks about steps to reach this goal. Which behavioral methods would likely work well?

   a. Shaping
   b. Punishment
   c. Tertiary intervention
   d. Tantrums

5. When Jillian, a 3-year-old, comes to her parents' room at night crying, her parents let her sleep with them. For Jillian's parents, this is an example of:

   a. Positive reinforcement
   b. Negative reinforcement
   c. Shaping
   d. Extinction

6. How should you encourage a parent to extinguish a behavior such as whining?

   a. Encourage the parent to spank the child for whining
   b. Encourage the parent to consistently ignore the whining behavior and give the child attention for desired behavior
   c. Encourage the parent to ignore everything the child does
   d. Encourage the parent to tell the child to stop whining in a calm voice

7. Elizabeth is at day care where she sees another child climb up on the counter to get a snack. Later that evening, Elizabeth attempts to climb the cabinets in her family's kitchen. Elizabeth learned this behavior through:

   a. Shaping
   b. Imitation

    c. Extinction

    d. Reinforcement

8. Which schedule of reinforcement is recommended if a child is learning a new skill?

    a. Fixed interval

    b. Variable interval

    c. Intermittent

    d. Continuous

9. Social Stories apply which behavioral principle:

    a. Modeling & Imitation

    b. Extinction

    c. Punishment

    d. Negative Reinforcement

10. Time Out is not generally an effective strategy for children who are?

    a. Less than 2 years old

    b. 3–8 years old

    c. Wanting to escape an aversive situation

    d. Both a and c

Assess Your Knowledge Answers
1) b   2) b   3) c   4) a   5) b   6) b   7) b   8) d   9) a   10) d

Chapter 7
Applying Principles of Behavior

Abstract This chapter outlines a process that early childhood professionals can use to address challenging behavior with behavioral strategies. The process begins with identifying a problem, considering why the problem is occurring, designing an intervention to address the problem, and using data to determine whether the intervention was effective in reducing the behavior and improving adaptive outcomes for the child.

Keywords Problem solving • ABC chart • Function of behavior • Triggers • Preventions • Replacement behavior

The Problem-Solving Process

Problem solving is used to define a problem and identify interventions which have the highest likelihood of improving outcomes. Problem solving focuses on identifying the specific behavioral issues a child is engaged in (e.g., hitting, swearing, whining) versus focusing on a description of a set of problems, or a diagnosis (e.g., tantrums or ADHD). Problem solving, when used in conjunction with the behavior principles, will help early intervention professionals develop interventions aimed to improve behavior and relationships, and teach new skills. The problem-solving process involves four steps, which are illustrated in Table 7.1.

Problem Identification

Problem identification involves 3 sub-steps described below:

Step 1. Define the problem behaviorally.
The first step involves describing the behavior in explicit terms, which is also referred to as the target behavior. Rather than indicating that a child has a tantrum,

K.H. Armstrong et al., *Evidence-Based Interventions for Children with Challenging Behavior*, DOI 10.1007/978-1-4614-7807-2_7, © Springer Science+Business Media New York 2014

Table 7.1 The problem-solving process

Problem identification *Is there a problem? What is it?*	A problem is defined as the discrepancy between the child's skills compared to other children or established benchmarks or milestones
Problem analysis *Why is the problem happening?*	Problem analysis involves trying to understand why the problem exists, applying the knowledge to formulate an effective plan of care, and selecting interventions with a high likelihood of success
Intervention implementation *What can be done about the problem?*	With successful problem analysis, a clearly defined intervention will become apparent. The plan should specify *who* will do *what*, *when* it will be done, and *how* long it will be tried. Also included in this plan is a data collection method to complete the fourth step
Intervention evaluation *Did the intervention work?*	This step involves examining the data and deciding whether the intervention needs to continue, be modified, or be discontinued

one would describe the behaviors composing the tantrum, such as falling to the floor, taking off and throwing a shoe, and crying so that the behavior becomes clearer to others. Several methods might be used to help identify the target behavior, such as observations, screening tools, and other assessments.

Step 2. Determine the replacement or desired behavior.
After specifically describing the problem behavior, one needs to identify the desired behavior, which is also referred to as the replacement behavior. The replacement behavior is the behavior that you want to replace the problem behavior, because it will make the child more successful if he or she is in a similar situation in the future. As with defining problem behaviors, replacement behaviors must be clearly defined. Replacement behaviors should lead to the development of new skills in a child, rather than just being something that would make things more convenient for the parent or teacher. For example, choosing "being silent" as a replacement behavior for crying and screaming when frustrated, might not address the fact that the child needs to learn more effective ways to communicate his or her frustration and ask for help. In this instance, teaching a child to use words or signs would be a more effective replacement skill for screaming. The early intervention professionals can pull from their knowledge of behavioral milestones, such as those outlined in Chap. 1, to determine what prosocial behavior might look like at different ages.

Step 3. Determine where the child's behavior falls in comparison to age expectations.
Once steps one and two are completed, the final step becomes easy. The early intervention professional determines where the child's behavior falls in comparison to expectations or benchmarks for children this age. This information is helpful in determining exactly how much growth is actually needed for the child to reach the desired goal. Should it become apparent that the child's behavior is not atypical, as compared with benchmarks, an early intervention professional would not need to conduct any further analyses, but instead would use this as an opportunity to provide anticipatory guidance to caregivers regarding development. In the case that a child's behavior was not consistent with established benchmarks, an early childhood professional would proceed to problem analysis.

Problem Analysis

After defining the behavior in relation to what is developmentally expected, the problem analysis stage is used to develop hypotheses to explain why the child is not exhibiting the desired behavior. It can be useful to think about risks that might be contributing to the problems, such as factors specific to the child (e.g., genetic and medical conditions, vision or hearing difficulties) as well as those in the child's environment (e.g., parenting practices, poverty, language use at home). For example, if a child comes to you because he or she is not using spoken words to communicate, there could be several reasons why the child is not talking. If the child cannot hear, he or she may not be talking. Alternatively, if no one talks to the child all day, and he or she sits in front of a television, the child also may not be talking. In either case, more information may be needed to understand the behavior, and to sort out what might be happening to maintain the behavior, in order to develop a clearly defined intervention plan. The goal at this stage is to develop a set of hypotheses related to why a child is exhibiting the target behavior or is unable to perform the replacement behavior.

A variety of methods can be used to collect data on what factors are contributing to a problem behavior, including interviews and observations. An ABC chart is a method that can be used to organize information about environmental factors that may be contributing to challenging behaviors. The ABC's of the ABC chart stand for *A*ntecedent, or the contexts surrounding the behavior such as who was present, what was happening, and when it occurred; *B*ehavior, or detailed description of the behavior; and *C*onsequence, or responses occurring after the behavior, which serve to maintain the behavior.

Figure 7.1 shows an example of an ABC-adapted chart taken from the Helping Our Toddlers, Developing Our Children's Skills Program (HOT DOCS; Armstrong, Lilly, Agazzi, & Williams 2010). In HOT DOCS, antecedents are referred to as "Triggers" and consequences as "Responses," to make it easier to comprehend. In addition, the HOT DOCS chart takes into account the *function* of the behavior, which is defined as the underlying motivation driving the behavior. Function may be simplified by determining what the behavior either helped the child to obtain or helped the child to escape. See Figure 7.2 for an example of the function of a behavior.

Once the behavior is clearly understood, the bottom half of the HOT DOCS chart can be used to document the interventions, and includes prevention strategies, new skills or replacement behaviors, and new responses which serve as reinforcers for the desired behavior, and consequences when the desired behavior does not happen. Figure 7.2 illustrates an example of determining the function of the behavior, based upon understanding triggers and consequences.

Another tool, the Functional Assessment Interview for Young Children (FAIYC; O'Neill et al., 1997), can provide very detailed information about complex behaviors that are not easily understood using approaches such as the ABC chart or the HOT DOCS chart. The FAIYC is a semi-structured caregiver interview, which also

Triggers	Behavior	Consequences
Describe events just before the behavior:	Specifically describe the behavior:	What happened following the behavior?
	Function? To GET or GET OUT OF:	
Preventions	**New Skills**	**New Responses**
What can be done to change or lessen the trigger(s)?	What skills are needed to perform the replacement behavior?	How will others now respond when the new behavior or problem behavior is displayed?

Fig. 7.1 HOT DOCS chart

Tony is a three year old with ASDs. He has a vocabulary limited to five words and two signs, which he uses inconsistently. Lately, Tony has begun hitting his mother, other children, and his daycare teacher. The hitting has become very frequent and he has hurt others. Tony hits when he does not want to do something, when he wants something, and sometimes he hits "playfully", perhaps wanting attention. After he hits, several different things happen as a consequence: he is sent to time out, he is given a drink, or he is picked up and told to "Stop it".

The HOT DOCS chart for Tony is summarized below:

Hypothesized Function	Triggers	Behavior	Consequences
Escape hand washing	Directed to wash hands	HITS	Put in Time Out and escapes hand washing
Wants drink	Sees mother at refrigerator	HITS	Mom looks down and gives him a drink
Wants attention	Sees peers in block area	HITS	Picked up by teacher and told to "Stop it."

Fig. 7.2 Function of behavior

collects observational data, to thoroughly (1) examine the environmental context related to the challenging behavior, (2) observe the child's communication strategies, and (3) help provide information about the function or conditions that account for the behavior.

Intervention Implementation

Based upon the information gathered through problem analysis, interventions are selected for implementation. The intervention should be tied to the hypothesis that is most likely to be the reason for the problem. If the analysis was successful, a clearly defined intervention will become apparent. For example, if it is hypothesized that Tony hits to get attention, an appropriate intervention would be to teach Tony another way to get attention from his teacher (e.g., raising his hand, pointing to a picture of what he wants) (see Fig. 7.3 for some examples). An early intervention professional might decide to develop an individual-specific intervention, based upon behavioral principles that are known to prevent, increase, or decrease behaviors or utilize an already developed intervention package, such as those discussed in Chap. 5. In designing or selecting interventions for young children, one must be mindful of the following issues:

- Is this intervention suitable for young children?
- Does the intervention present unnecessary risks?
- Does the intervention require too much caregiver time?
- Does the intervention have negative side effects on other children in the family or in the classroom?
- Does the caregiver have the motivation and skills to implement the intervention?
- Does this intervention respect the cultural values of the family?

Intervention Evaluation

The last phase of problem solving with behavioral strategies involves evaluating the intervention that was developed to address the problem. This step is essential to ensure that the intervention is not only implemented, but that it is resulting in a positive outcome for the child and their family. Simple data collection procedures must be included in any intervention plan and will be discussed in more depth in Chap. 8. This process is often referred to as progress monitoring, because the data are used to document the intervention process.

Finally, any time an intervention plan is developed, the team should specify a timeframe to review the progress of the intervention. The data used to monitor the

Problem Solving: Building New Skills

Bryan is a two year-old boy whose primary behavior concern is excessive tantrums. Through problem identification and problem analysis, the following information is generated:

- **Problem Identification:** Bryan tantrums 10 times a day, defined as screaming, throwing toys, crying, and laying down on the floor, and banging his head so hard that he has bruises. These episodes last from 20-35 minutes. The intensity and duration of the episodes make this behavior atypical. The desired replacement behavior is that Bryan will request more time when he does not want to stop an activity
- **Problem Analysis:** The tantrums are more likely to occur at home and during times where Bryan must transition from something he likes, such as playing with his toys, to something he does not like as much, like riding in the car to do errands. The early childhood professional and Bryan's mother think that their most valid hypothesis to explain Bryan's tantrums is that he wants to play longer and he often avoids the car ride and errands. In addition, he lacks the skills to ask for more time or tell his mother that he does not want to stop playing. More than 50% of the time, Bryan's mother gives in to Bryan; they stay home where he can continue to play. She sometimes uses time out, or picks him up and puts him in his car seat, depending on the time of day. The function of his behavior is to communicate "I do not want to stop playing."

To address this concern, the early childhood professional and parent agree to implement an intervention plan, the goal of which will be to teach Bryan to ask for "more play time" rather than screaming. To reinforce the use of this new skill, Bryan's mother will prompt him to request "more play time", and will allow him to play for "5 more minutes", and set a timer to signal the interval, and let him know when play time is over. If Bryan whined or cried, he would be prompted again to say "more play time", and given a few seconds to comply. All challenging behavior would be ignored, and cooperation praised. The end goal would be to eliminate the frequency of tantrums by teaching Bryan to use words for requests.

Problem Solving: Shaping New Behaviors

William is a two-year-old boy who does not use words when he is with his parents. Although he has been enrolled in speech and is progressing with the therapist, he is not using words at home. To communicate his needs at home, William may hit a parent, shriek, or begin crying. William's mother, Tina, will often give in to William, to end the behavior problems, and is becoming increasingly less tolerant.

- **Problem Identification:** William will cry, shriek, or hit his mother throughout the day when he needs something. William has demonstrated a vocabulary and gestures appropriate for his age when working with the therapist such as pointing, or naming the object. The desired replacement behavior is for William to use his words at home.
- **Problem Analysis:** An ABC Chart was completed when William showed problem behaviors. Results showed that in almost 70% of the instances where William used one of his problem behaviors, Tina gave him what he wanted. It was hypothesized that this reinforced the use of these behaviors.

Tina and the early childhood professional determine that William needs to communicate his needs verbally at home. To accomplish this, Tina will offer him limited choices, model words for William and immediately reinforce any attempts to communicate with praise and the item he wants. At first, all verbal attempts are reinforced, and then upon consultation with the early childhood professional, Tina will gradually reinforce only attempts which are closer to the target word. She will also ignore any unwanted behaviors. Tina is to prompt William by saying "use your words" and provide enthusiastic attention for approximations toward the use of words.

Fig. 7.3 Examples of application of problem solving utilizing behavioral strategies. Presents examples of how early childhood professionals use problem-solving with parents and caregivers

Problem Solving: Using Social Stories

Laura is four-years-old and has been diagnosed with ASDs. A primary concern to Laura's mom, Diana, is that she cannot take Laura to the library and have her exhibit appropriate behavior. When going to the library, Laura tries to run away from Diana, screams, and lays down on the floor.

- **Problem Identification:** Laura does not display appropriate behaviors when entering the library with her mother. Instead she resists and engages in multiple behaviors to delay or prevent Diana and her from entering the library. The desired replacement behavior is that Laura holds her mother's hand to enter the library, and that she use words or pictures to express herself.

- **Problem Analysis:** After completing an FAIYC, the early childhood professional and Diana think that Laura becomes overwhelmed by several aspects of the library and tries to leave because she is uncomfortable in that situation. It is also possible that Laura does not have some of the skills needed to be in the library such as speaking quietly.

To address these problematic behaviors, Diana and the early childhood professional develop a social story which Diana reads several times a day with Laura. The story helps to prepare Laura for this experience by telling her what is going to happen, how she should behave, how she will feel, and how others will feel when she makes these good choices. In addition, they practice at home all of the skills included within the story such as entering the library, walking while in the library, choosing a book, and speaking in a whisper. As Laura masters specific skills, Diana takes her to the library and coaches Laura in these steps, using ample praise and rewards. Eventually, Laura becomes comfortable with the library and is able to remain calm when they visit it.

Problem Solving: Using Time Out

Lilly is a three-year old girl who refuses to comply when told to clean up her toys. She ignores her mother's directions, continues playing, and may even begin whining. Her mother pleads with her to clean up the toys, saying "Can't you pick up your toys?" Lilly responds by throwing her toys at her mother. This behavior happens several times over the course of the day, and Lilly's mother is quite frustrated.

- **Problem Identification:** Lilly throwing toys at her mother when she is asked to clean up, and this occurs several times per day. The desired replacement behavior is for Lilly to follow her mother's directions to clean up toys within 20 seconds.

- **Problem Analysis:** These episodes are more likely to occur at home and during times when Lilly must transition to another activity that she may not enjoy. Using the HOT DOCS Chart, the early intervention professional and Lilly's mother decide that the function of the behavior is to escape, so Lilly misbehaves so that she can play longer. This behavior is maintained because Lilly gets to play longer, her mother eventually gives in, and may even pick up the toys herself.

To address this behavior, Lilly's mother is taught to give Lilly an effective command with a transition warning, "In 5 minutes, you will need to clean up your toys." Five minutes pass, signaled by the timer, and Lilly's mother says, "Please clean up your toys." If Lilly complies, her mother praises her. If not, her mother repeats the command, and informs Lilly that if she does not clean up her toys, she will go to the time out chair. If Lilly still does not follow this direction, her mother leads her to the time out chair and says "you did not clean up your toys when I asked you to, so you will have to sit in the time out chair. Stay here until I tell you that you can get up". Her Mother walks away, and waits for 3 minutes. She returns to Lilly and says "You are sitting quietly. Are you ready to clean your toys up now?" If Lilly says yes, she is directed to the toys, and mother acknowledges her efforts by saying "thank you for listening". If Lilly does not do this, the time out process starts again. After a few times of using this procedure, Lilly learns to follow her mother's directions because the process is clear, and she does not want to sit in time out.

Fig. 7.3 (continued)

intervention progress will make it clear whether the intervention should be continued, discontinued, or modified. Figure 7.3 presents examples of how early childhood professionals use problem-solving with parents and caregivers.

Conclusions

This chapter describes the problem-solving process with the use of behavioral technology in designing and implementing interventions to address problem behavior and improve developmental functioning. The skillful use of the problem-solving model along with behavioral technology will help to articulate the problem, determine how to address the problem, and evaluate whether the intervention plan was successful in addressing the presenting concerns. As such, the resulting intervention plan will be based upon the best evidence available, and valuable time and resources will be wisely spent. The next chapters will detail the process of using data for progress monitoring to document the response to intervention.

Assess Your Knowledge

Use the questions below to assess your knowledge of the information presented in this chapter. Answers appear after the last question.

1. Which of the following factors should be considered when developing your hypotheses about why a behavior is occurring?

   a. Child
   b. Family
   c. Community
   d. All of the above

2. Which of the following is <u>NOT</u> a good definition of a child's problematic behavior?

   a. Spitting
   b. Biting another child
   c. Having a hissy fit
   d. Laying on floor, arms hitting floor, and screaming for at least 2 min

3. When designing an intervention for a child, which of the following questions are most important to keep in mind?

   a. Does the caregiver have the skills to implement it?
   b. Will the child like the intervention?
   c. How will other people view the child's behavior?
   d. Can other people assist with the intervention?

4. To assist with the Problem Analysis step, one can use:

   a. An ABC chart
   b. The HOT DOCS chart
   c. Behavior ratings
   d. All options are correct

5. The four problem-solving steps include:

   a. Problem Identification, Problem Analysis, Intervention Implementation, Intervention Evaluation
   b. Problem Focus, Problem Analysis, Intervention Planning, Intervention Implementation
   c. Problem Identification, Intervention Planning, Intervention Analysis, Evaluation
   d. Problem, Naming the Problem, Intervention Planning, Intervention Analysis

6. What are the sub-steps within the Problem Identification stage?

   a. Define a problem, develop expectations for age, measure differences in child's skills
   b. Define the problem behaviorally, define a new behavior, compare a child's performance to baseline
   c. Define the problem behaviorally, establish the desired level of behavior, compare a child's performance with age expectations
   d. Define a problem, define a new behavior, compare a child's performance with age expectations

7. In developing an intervention, it is essential to understand the following:

   a. Child's preferences for intervention
   b. Child's diagnosis
   c. Function of the behavior
   d. Both a & b

8. Hypotheses about why the behavior occurs are generated during which stage?

   a. Problem Identification
   b. Problem Analysis
   c. Intervention Implementation
   d. Intervention Evaluation

9. The problem-solving process can stop when:

   a. The problem identification stage shows the child is not behind his or her peers in development
   b. The first intervention is completed
   c. Problem analysis is finished
   d. No intervention can be developed for a problem

10. If the problem has not been resolved by the end of the problem-solving process, one should:

    a. Immediately stop the current intervention
    b. Revisit the problem identification step and begin the process again
    c. Try a new intervention
    d. Refer the child to a different practitioner

Assess Your Knowledge Answers
1) d   2) c   3) a   4) d   5) a   6) a   7) c   8) b   9) a   10) b

Chapter 8
Progress Monitoring

Abstract Monitoring a child's progress toward a predetermined goal is critical in ensuring the effectiveness of intervention. This chapter describes the importance of progress monitoring as it relates to the problem-solving process, explains the various methods of tracking progress, and guides practitioners in the selection of appropriate progress monitoring tools.

Keywords Response to intervention • Problem solving • Rating scales • Behavioral observation • General outcome measurements • Individual growth and developmental indicators for infants and toddlers • Naturalistic observation • Systematic direct observation

Introduction to Progress Monitoring

Engaging in evidence-based practice means that providers select interventions because of the benefit they offer to targeted problems. However, implementing evidence-based interventions does not guarantee desired outcomes. Therefore, progress must be monitored in order to evaluate whether an intervention is working as intended.

Progress monitoring refers to the practice of using data to measure growth toward a specified goal. This process helps us to answer such questions as, "Is this program or intervention working?", "Has the child gained skills since the last assessment?", or "Does the child require additional or different interventions?". If the data reveals positive change, there is evidence for continuing the intervention. If the data display no change or negative change, the intervention should be adjusted. Progress monitoring ensures that valuable resources are not wasted on ineffective interventions, and that children do not fall further behind as a result.

Progress monitoring data can be captured using an existing tool or practitioners can design a progress monitoring method specific to the targeted concern. Regardless

Table 8.1 Using the problem-solving process

Case study: Ethan	
Background information	
Ethan is not talking yet, even though he is almost 3 years old	
Problem identification	Comparing Ethan's speech and language skills to language milestones suggests a delay. He has a vocabulary of about 10–15 words, shows little interest in imitating sounds, and does not answer to his name. He is unable to follow one-step commands without prompting
Problem analysis	Audiology results indicate that Ethan has normal hearing for speech sounds. Developmental assessment indicates significant delays in receptive and expressive language skills, but otherwise typical development. An oral-motor exam was also normal. The assessment team decides that Ethan needs help to improve receptive and expressive skills
Intervention implementation	The picture exchange communication system (PECS) is an augmentative communication system developed to help children who do not use speech or who may speak with limited effectiveness, quickly acquire a functional means of communication (Bondy & Frost, 1994). Parents and the interventionist work together to identify Ethan's preferences, and begin to implement this intervention at home and in other settings. They will teach Ethan to point to pictures for requests. Pointing is immediately praised by the caregiver, who also models the spoken word for the request
Progress monitoring	Parent and interventionist both tally the number of requests Ethan makes using pictures. New pictures are added as Ethan expands his vocabulary. Eventually, Ethan's use of spoken words for requests will be tallied

of the method, progress monitoring data documents the development of new skills over a period of time. These new skills are often referred to as replacement skills or desired behaviors. Along with tracking desired behavior, progress monitoring measures the reduction of the undesirable or problematic behavior. For example, an intervention may be designed to improve a child's bedtime habits. To progress monitor the effectiveness of this intervention, a parent may record the number of minutes it takes the child to stop crying after being put to bed (e.g., reduction of the undesirable behavior) as well as the total hours that the child sleeps without waking (e.g., increase in desired behavior or new skills). Data can also be collected to track changes in an adult's behavior. For example, a parent might be asked to document the number of positive statements he or she uses to encourage his or her child's prosocial behavior. By tallying this number and graphing the data, he or she can see if his or her use of positive statements is increasing.

Progress monitoring tools are different from screening instruments or comprehensive assessments. Progress monitoring tools measure only specific skills and serve as indicators of growth toward a predetermined outcome or goal. Because we want to track the development of new skills, it is ideal to measure both the undesirable and desired behavior. However, if it is feasible to measure only one behavior it is recommended that the replacement behavior be progress monitored. An example of how progress monitoring is incorporated within the problem-solving process appears in Table 8.1.

Progress Monitoring Methods

There are several ways to monitor whether a child is exhibiting a particular behavior. These include commercial rating scales and individual behavioral observations. These two broad methods of progress monitoring are described in the following sections.

Rating Scales

Commercial rating scales rely on parent or caregiver reports of the frequency or intensity of a child's behavior. Rating scales typically describe specific behaviors and require a person to answer whether or not a child exhibits that behavior. For example, one question on a rating scale may be, "Does the child follow one step commands during play?" Rating scales often ask parents to rate how frequently a behavior occurs. For example, a parent may be asked to respond to the question posed previous ("Does the child follow one step commands during play?") with "never," "sometimes," "often," or "very often." Rating scales can be completed by the parent independently or through an interview between the examiner and the parent, and the child need not be present during the administration. These instruments are particularly useful when considering that some child behaviors might not occur outside of the family setting (e.g., toilet training, sleeping habits). However, since rating scales are based on parental report, the accuracy of the data depends on whether the parent was present when the behavior occurred as well their memory of the child's behavior. Therefore, it is important to ask the parent or person who spends the most time with the child to complete items to ensure the most accurate data.

The Ages and Stages Questionnaire: Social Emotional (ASQ-SE) and Assessment, Evaluation, and Programming System for Infants and Children-Second Edition (AEPS) are examples of commercially produced rating scales that may be appropriate for progress monitoring, and are described below.

Ages and Stages Questionnaire: Social Emotional (ASQ-SE)			
Domain and goal:	Social/emotional development (i.e., self-regulation, compliance, communication, adaptive behaviors, autonomy, affect, and interaction with people)	For:	3–66 months of age
Type:	Rating scale	Length:	10–15 min to administer 2–3 min to score
Description:	The ASQ-SE can be used as a screener and/or for progress monitoring. There are 8 different parent questionnaires spanning across the age range		
Strengths:	Available in Spanish; simple and easy to follow (Vacca, 2005)	Limitations:	Generalizability of scores across gender, race, and ethnicity is unknown (Vacca, 2012)

Assessment, Evaluation, and Programming System (AEPS) for Infants and Children (Second Edition)

Domain and goal:	Motor skills, adaptive functioning, cognitive development, communication, and social/emotional development	For:	Birth to 6 years old
Type:	Observation and/or rating scale	Length:	1–2 h for initial assessment, 15–30 minutes for subsequent assessments
Description:	A criterion-referenced tool that evaluates a child's developmental progress of functional skills across the different domains. Each domain is divided into discrete objectives or skills leading up to specific goals for that domain. Based on parent report, observation, or direct elicitation of skills from the child, the examiner records whether the child consistently performs, inconsistently performs, or does not perform the skills. Can be re-administered at 3- or 4-month intervals		
Strengths:	Complete systematic assessment has direct links to intervention planning (Bagnato, Neisworth, & Munson, 1997; Horn, 2003; as cited in Van Haneghan, 2009). Can be re-administered at 3- or 4-month intervals	Limitations:	Initial entire assessment can be time-consuming to administer and expertise in assessment domains is recommended (Van Haneghan, 2009)

Behavioral Observations

Progress monitoring can also be performed by directly observing a child's behavior. There are a number of different methods of observing behavior. Some methods are more informal and entail writing down everything one observes in a narrative format. Other behavioral observation methods are more systematic and include carefully specified procedures. For example, one might document the number of 10 seconds intervals during which a child was actively watching the teacher or following along in class. This type of behavioral observation is often referred to as systematic direct observations (SDO) and is more reliable than narrative recording of a child's behavior. These methods will be discussed in more detail later in this chapter. Additionally, there are already-made tools available for behavioral observations or practitioners can create their own. Both types are described below.

Existing Tools

Several observation tools are already available for progress monitoring the development of young children. Although it can be helpful to progress monitor one specific behavior (such as a child's hours of sleep per night or number of spoken words), it may be even more valuable to measure a child's progress toward important developmental outcomes. General Outcome Measurements (GOMs) are progress monitoring assessments used to evaluate growth toward key developmental skills. GOMs are unique in that these tools are sensitive to improved performance on the same developmental skills, rather than simply whether or not a child has achieved mastery on a number of different skills. Individual Growth and Developmental Indicators for Infants and Toddlers (IGDIs) are examples of GOMs designed for young children (Walker, Cartta, Greenwood, & Buzhardt 2008). Preschool IGDIs are also available. The IGDIs include a coding system and graphing to progress monitor skills in developmental domains.

IGDIs are available for use for the following domains of development: adaptive functioning, communication, motor skills, cognitive development, and social/emotional development. The following are examples of IGDIs that may be used to progress monitor a child's early development in different areas.

Early Problem-Solving Indicator (EPSI; Greenwood, Walker, Carta, & Higgins, 2006)			
Domain and goal:	Cognitive development: "Child solves problems that require reasoning about objects, concepts, situations, and people"	For:	Birth to 4 years
Type:	Observation	Length:	6 min
Description:	During administration of the EPSI, an adult familiar to the child engages in play with the child and one of the three toys selected to evoke problem-solving behaviors from the child (i.e., a pop-up toy, stacking toys, and a drop tower). The adult presents each toy for 2 min (for a total administration time of 6 min) while another adult records the child's behavior by observing how the child interacts with the toys and whether he or she uses the toys for his or her intended purposes. Key skill elements consist of *look* (looking at the toy), *explore* (manipulating, rubbing, touching, etc., the toy), *function* (making the toy perform its intended function), and *solution* (engaging in a fluid sequence of skills with a toy leading to its intended objective)		
Strengths:	Administration and scoring materials and training documents are available free of charge on the IGDIs Web site	Limitations:	Not yet reviewed
Web site:	http://www.igdi.ku.edu/index.htm		

Early Communication Indicator (ECI; Greenwood, Carta, Walker, Hughes, & Weathers, 2006)			
Domain and goal:	Communication: child's expressive communication skills including gestures, vocalizations, single-word, and multiple-word utterances	For:	Birth to 3 years
Type:	Observation	Length:	6 min for administration
Description:	The ECI involves play between the child, a familiar adult, and a toy. The adult's play should encourage the child to interact with the toy and the adult. A second adult observes and scores the interactions by tallying the frequency of gestures, vocalizations, single-word, and multiple-word utterances made by the child, or the administration can be videotaped for later scoring		

(continued)

(continued)

Early Communication Indicator (ECI; Greenwood, Carta, Walker, Hughes, & Weathers, 2006)

Strengths:	Accommodations can be made for children with sensory/physical problems and for Spanish-speakers; administration and scoring materials and training documents are available free of charge on the IGDIs Web site	Limitations:	Not yet reviewed
Web site:	http://www.igdi.ku.edu/index.htm		

Early Movement Indicator (EMI; Greenwood, Luze, Cline, Kuntz, & Leitschuh, 2002)

Domain and goal:	Motor skills: "The child moves in a fluent and coordinated manner to play and participate in home, school, and community settings"	For:	Birth to 3 years
Type:	Observation	Length:	6 min
Description:	EMI administration involves a familiar adult engaging the child in play with a toy intended to evoke movement from the child. A second adult records the child's movement by coding the key skills (transitional movements, grounded locomotion, vertical locomotion, throwing/rolling, catching/trapping) the child demonstrates		
Strengths:	Administration and scoring materials and training documents are available free of charge on the IGDIs Web site	Limitations:	Not yet reviewed
Web site:	http://www.igdi.ku.edu/index.htm		

Early Social Indicator (ESI; Carta, Greenwood, Luze, Cline, & Kuntz, 2004)

Domain and goal:	Social/emotional development: "Child interacts with peers and adults, maintaining social interaction and participating socially in home, school, and community"	For:	Birth to 3 years
Type:	Observation	Length:	6 min
Description:	The ECI consists of an adult (familiar to the child), child, and a child's peer to engage with different toys for 6 min while another adult codes and scores the child's behavior. ECI key skill elements vary across three dimensions: verbal/nonverbal communication, target of communication (adult or peer), and positive/negative interaction		
Strengths:	Administration and scoring materials and training documents are available free of charge on the IGDIs Web site	Limitations:	Not yet reviewed
Web site:	http://www.igdi.ku.edu/index.htm		

Indicator of Parent–Child Interaction (IPCI; Baggett & Carta, 2006)

Domain and goal:	Parent interaction: child interactions with caregivers should promote positive child social-emotional behaviors	For:	Birth to 3 years
Type:	Observation	Length:	8–10 min

(continued)

(continued)

Indicator of Parent–Child Interaction (IPCI; Baggett & Carta, 2006)			
Description:	The IPCI is a progress monitoring tool for evaluating parent and child interactions in response to an intervention. IPCI administration involves a parent interacting with the child in common activities, such as free play, book reading, dressing, and a distraction test. During these interactions, behaviors in four domains are documented: parent/caregiver supporting behavior, parent/caregiver interrupting behavior, child engagement, and child reactivity/distress		
Strengths:	Administration and scoring materials and training documents are available free of charge on the IGDIs Web site	Limitations:	Not yet reviewed
Web site:	http://www.igdi.ku.edu/index.htm		

General Outcome Measurements for Preschool

The following IGDIs were designed to assess and monitor the progress of emerging literacy skills and are appropriate for children 3–5 years of age. These IGDIs tap skills in vocabulary and phonemic awareness, which are predictors of later reading achievement.

Picture Naming (McConnell, McEvoy, & Priest, 2002)			
Domain and goal:	Vocabulary (early literacy)	For:	Three to five years of age
Type:	Observation	Length:	2 min to both administer and score
Description:	The examiner presents the child with different pictures of common items found at home, school, and the community one at a time. The child is asked to name the pictures as fast as possible. The examiner counts the total number of correctly identified pictures after that 1 min		
Strengths:	Clear scoring guidelines; colorful and appealing materials; user-friendly Web site (Wackerle, 2007)	Limitations:	Some responses to items may not be accepted as correct (e.g., "sofa" is incorrect for a picture of a couch; Wackerle, 2007)
Web site:	http://www.myigdis.com/		

Alliteration (McConnell, Priest, Davis, & McEvoy, 2002)			
Domain and goal:	Phonemic awareness (early literacy)	For:	Three to five years of age
Type:	Observation	Length:	3 min to both administer and score

(continued)

(continued)

Alliteration (McConnell, Priest, Davis, & McEvoy, 2002)			
Description:	The examiner shows the child a picture of a common word and then shows three other pictures. The child is asked to point to which of the three other pictures starts with the same sound as the first picture. After 2 minutes, the examiner totals how many pictures the child correctly identified		
Strengths:	Clear scoring guidelines; colorful and appealing materials; user-friendly Web site (Wackerle, 2007)	Limitations:	Some items may be somewhat obsolete for today's children (e.g., illustration of jacks and a ball; Wackerle, 2007)
Web site:	http://www.myigdis.com/		

Rhyming (McConnell et al., 2002)			
Domain and goal:	Phonemic awareness (early literacy)	For:	3–5 years of age
Type:	Observation	Length:	Approximately 3 min to both administer and score
Description:	The examiner shows the child a picture of a common word and then shows three other pictures. The child is asked to point to which of the three other pictures sounds the same as (or rhymes with) the first picture. After 2 minutes, the examiner totals how many pictures the child correctly identified		
Strengths:	Clear scoring guidelines; colorful and appealing materials; user-friendly Web site (Wackerle, 2007)	Limitations:	Some items may be somewhat obsolete for today's children (e.g., illustration of jacks and a ball; Wackerle, 2007)
Web site:	http://www.myigdis.com/		

Creating Your Own Progress Monitoring Tool

As is often the case in early intervention, a practitioner may find that they need to design a progress monitoring tool specific to the unique needs presented by the child and caregivers. There are generally two observation techniques that one can employ for progress monitoring of specific behaviors: naturalistic observation and systematic direct observations. Both methods are described below.

Naturalistic Observation

A narrative recording is an informal naturalistic observation. Narrative recording involves writing down everything observed to create a descriptive, time-sequenced account of all behaviors. Particular attention is paid to the target behaviors and anything that happens before (antecedents) and after (consequences) the target behavior occurs. This detailed narrative can then be analyzed to identify the pattern of behavior leading up to and following the target behavior.

To conduct a narrative recording, follow these four steps:

1. Set aside a 20–30 min period to continuously observe the child. Have several sheets of paper and a writing utensil. Try to be as unobtrusive as possible to avoid the child behaving differently than normal because he or she is being observed.
2. Write down everything the child does and says and everything that happens to the child. Only the observed behaviors should be recorded, not interpretations of behaviors. It can also be helpful to make notes of relevant aspects of the environment (e.g., number of children or adults present and their placement). The following is an excerpt of a narrative recording:

> Ethan stacks up colored blocks on top of one another. Ethan says to his mom, "Look." Ethan's mom looks at Ethan and says, "Good job, Ethan. What are those called?" Ethan says, "Blocks." Ethan's mom smiles and says, "That's right! They are blocks. What color is this one?" Ethan's mom picks up a green block. Ethan says, "Green!" Ethan's mom smiles and says, "Good boy! This one is green. What color is this one?" Ethan's mom holds up a yellow block. Ethan pauses. Ethan says, "Blue." Ethan's mom says, "No, this is not a blue block, Ethan. Try again. What color is this block?" Ethan says, "Yellow?" Ethan's mom smiles and says, "Yes! Good job!"

3. After the observation period is over, the narrative can be organized into Antecedents (what happened before a behavior), Behavior, and Consequences (what happened after a behavior). A chart is often useful for this purpose. The ABC chart is focused on the child's behavior. Also keep in mind that the consequence of one behavior may serve as the antecedent of the next behavior. Table 8.2 below shows how the above narrative recording would be put into an ABC chart (Sample in Appendix B, C):
4. By looking at this ABC Chart, one can identify antecedents/triggers or what happens before Ethan says a word, and consequences or responses from others that are reinforcing the behavior. From analyzing this chart, one could hypothesize that Ethan's use of words is reinforced by his mother's attention (looking, descriptive words, praise, etc.), and in addition, more words are prompted by his mother's interactions.

Narrative recordings can be a very useful observation technique, particularly for understanding why a behavior is occurring by looking at factors that may trigger and reinforce the behavior. This observation technique allows the observer not only to record the child's behavior but also to consider the environmental factors that

Table 8.2 Example ABC chart

Antecedent (A)	Behavior (B)	Consequence (C)
Ethan stacks up colored blocks on top of one another	Ethan says to his mom, "Look"	Ethan's mom looks at Ethan and says, "Good job, Ethan. What are those called?"
Ethan's mom looks at Ethan and says, "Good job, Ethan. What are those called?"	Ethan says, "Blocks"	Ethan's mom smiles and says, "That's right! They are blocks. What color is this one?" Ethan's mom picks up a green block
Ethan's mom smiles and says, "That's right! They are blocks. What color is this one?" Ethan's mom picks up a green block	Ethan says, "Green!"	Ethan's mom smiles and says, "Good boy! This one is green. What color is this one?" Ethan's mom holds up a yellow block
Ethan's mom smiles and says, "Good boy! This one is green. What color is this one?" Ethan's mom holds up a yellow block	Ethan pauses. Ethan says, "Blue"	Ethan's mom says, "No, this is not a blue block, Ethan. Try again. What color is this block?"
Ethan's mom says, "No, this is not a blue block, Ethan. Try again. What color is this block?"	Ethan says, "Yellow?"	Ethan's mom smiles and says, "Yes! Good job!"

contribute to the target behavior. As such, this type of observation is often used during the problem analysis phase of problem solving in order to collect more information about why a problem is occurring. Although this observation method may be useful when progress monitoring in some circumstances, it may not be the most efficient method of observation for progress monitoring purposes. Specifically, narrative observation can be more time-consuming than other observation methods and it can also be difficult to quantify the behaviors observed during a narrative recording. In other words, it can be challenging to systematically compare multiple narrative observations making it difficult to objectively evaluate progress toward a goal.

Systematic Direct Observations

Systematic Direct Observations (SDO) offer a more precise account of progress toward a goal. Generally speaking, SDO involves observing and recording whether or not a specific behavior occurs. To conduct an SDO the desired behavior must first be identified. As described in previous chapters, the behavioral description for a target behavior must be clear, specific, and complete. Because behaviors can be described and measured in several different ways, or dimensions, the particular dimension of behavior to measure should be selected. Commonly used dimensions that can measure behavior include count, frequency/rate, duration, magnitude, and latency. Please see Table 8.3 for definitions and examples of each dimension.

When behaviors occur continuously or on a very frequent basis, tallying the occurrence of every single instance of the behavior may not be feasible. Fortunately,

Table 8.3 Common dimensions of behavior

	Definition	Behavioral example	Example with Ethan
Count	The number of occurrences of a behavior	The number of bites of food a child eats at dinner	Ethan's mother counts the number of words Ethan utters each day
Frequency/rate	The number of occurrences of a behavior within a specific amount of time	The number of labeled praises a parent uses in 15 min	Practitioner observes Ethan and mother play and counts number of labeled praises used in 15 min
Duration	The amount of time a behavior occurs	The number of hours a child sleeps each night	Ethan's mother documents the number of hours Ethan sleeps each night over a week
Magnitude/intensity	The intensity or force with which a behavior is produced	The loudness of a child's vocalizations (i.e., mumbling versus talking loudly)	Ethan's mother rates the volume of Ethan's speech on a rating scale from 0 to 5
Latency	The elapsed time between a prompt and a behavioral response	Number of seconds between an adult's command ("Pick up your toys") and the child's compliance	Ethan's mother records the time it takes for Ethan to respond to this direct command

there are observation methods that do not require measuring the count, duration, etc., of each instance of the behavior. Instead, these methods involve collecting samples of behavior to estimate its occurrence. Time sampling involves observing and recording behavior during specific moments in time (referred to as intervals). In time sampling, an observation period is divided up into time intervals (before the observation begins) and then the practitioner records whether or not the behavior occurred for each interval (Cooper, Heron, & Heward, 2007). Table 8.4 details the guidelines for selecting a method.

Conclusions

Considering the variety of progress monitoring methods and tools available, it is necessary to carefully consider the options before collecting data. It is important to note that while creating your own system for tracking progress is helpful, it is also valuable to use GOMs to track the child's progress toward developmental milestones. Both of these tools can be used together.

Table 8.4 Time sampling observation methods

	Definition	When most useful	Example with Ethan
Whole interval time sampling	Records the behavior only when it is emitted throughout the entire interval	Useful when it is important to know that the behavior is not interrupted. Tends to underestimate occurrences of behavior	Break up an hour into ten 6 min intervals. During each interval, record whether or not Ethan speaks the *entire* 10 min interval
Partial interval time sampling	Records the behavior when a single instance of the behavior occurs in the interval. Tends to overestimate the occurrence of the behavior	Used to record behaviors that may occur in fleeting moments	Break up an hour into ten 6 min intervals. During each interval, record whether Ethan says at *least* one word for each interval
Momentary time sampling	Records the behavior if emitted at the moment the interval begins	Tends to be the most accurate time sampling method	Break up an hour into ten 6 min intervals. Either at the start or end of each 10 min interval, record if Ethan is speaking *right at that moment*

In selecting progress monitoring tools, the following three features should be taken into account: authenticity, utility, and universality (Bagnato, 2006). To be *authentic*, a measurement tool must involve natural, everyday routines and activities in a familiar, and everyday environment (e.g., home or daycare) with a familiar and knowledgeable person (e.g., parent, teacher) observing. *Utility* refers to the purpose of measurement tools. A measurement tool should assess a child's skills and then use the results to develop and evaluate goals and interventions. *Universality* maintains that assessment tools should be functional and flexible enough to be applied to all children.

Assess Your Knowledge

Use the questions below to assess your knowledge of the information presented in this chapter. Answers appear after the last question.

1. Which of the following is NOT a reason you would want to progress monitor a child's behavior after implementing an intervention?

   a. So you know whether or not your intervention is working
   b. To ensure you are not wasting time and money on an ineffective intervention

    c. It allows you to know when the intervention is no longer needed or could be reduced

    d. It tells you why an intervention is not working

2. Progress monitoring tools:

    a. Are comprehensive

    b. Are time-consuming

    c. Measure progress toward a specific goal

    d. Are very difficult to create

3. Rating scales are particularly helpful for behaviors that:

    a. Are not easily observable outside of the family.

    b. Are easily observable by a member outside of the family

    c. Occurred a long time ago

    d. Occur many times throughout the day.

4. During a naturalistic observation, you would:

    a. Mark every third time a behavior occurs.

    b. Record the duration of each behavior.

    c. Write down exactly what is occurring.

    d. Rate how intense a behavior is

5. Which of the following is NOT a dimension of behavior?

    a. Rate

    b. Frequency

    c. Duration

    d. Event recording

6. If you kept track of the number of times a child swore, you would be using which dimension to measure behavior?

    a. Count

    b. Latency

    c. Duration

    d. Magnitude

7. You want a parent to record how many seconds it takes for a child to comply with a request, which dimension of behavior is this?

    a. Count

    b. Latency

    c. Duration

    d. Magnitude

8. With whole interval time sampling

    a. You record whether a behavior occurs throughout an entire interval

    b. You record whether a behavior occurs at all during an interval

    c. You record whether a behavior occurs only at the start of the interval
    d. You record whether a behavior occurs only at the end of the interval

9. When examining an assessment for use with children, which of the following is NOT an important feature?

    a. Efficiency
    b. Utility
    c. Universality
    d. Authenticity

10. A primary concern for Bryce's parents is that he rarely has tantrums but when he does, they last for over 45 min. If you are implementing an intervention to reduce his tantrums, what dimension of behavior should you measure?

    a. Count
    b. Frequency
    c. Magnitude
    d. Duration

Assess Your Knowledge Answers
1) d   2) c   3) a   4) c   5) d   6) a   7) b   8) b   9) c   10) d

Chapter 9
Evaluating Outcomes

Abstract The final step in the problem-solving process is to evaluate the effectiveness of the intervention. One way to make data more easily interpretable is to display it visually. By graphing data both providers and caregivers are able to see changes in the behavior measured and decisions about interventions can be made. Graphs can be created through drawing by hand or using computer programs, such as Microsoft Excel.

Keywords Baseline data • Intervention data • *X*-axis • *Y*-axis • Phase change line • Continuing an intervention • Modifying an intervention • Discontinuing an intervention

Once progress monitoring data has been collected for a minimum of three different points, this data should be plotted on a graph. Visual displays provide a simple way to quickly interpret progress monitoring data and determine whether or not an intervention has been effective. Graphs require little time to create once you understand the basic components. Graphs can be created by hand or through computer programs such as Microsoft Excel. In the following sections, both graphing methods will be described.

Important Graphing Terms

- *Baseline Data*: Baseline data refers to the data collected about a behavior prior to intervention. When one looks at data of a behavior before and after intervention implementation, they are able to infer about the intervention's impact. (A in graph below)
- *Intervention Data*: Intervention data refers to the data collected after an intervention has been put into place. Intervention data allows one to see if the behavior has changed after intervention implementation. (B in graph below)

- *X-Axis*: The horizontal axis of the graph represents the time the data was collected. This axis could be divided into minutes, hours, days, weeks, and so on. For example, if the number of hours a child sleeps each night were being measured, the X-Axis would represent night of the week. (C in graph)
- *Y-Axis*: The vertical axis of the graph represents the instances of a behavior. This axis could be divided into number of times the behavior occurs, number of minutes, and so forth. For example, if one was measuring the number of hours a child sleeps each night, the Y-Axis would represent number of hours of sleep. (D in graph)
- *Phase Change Line*: A vertical, dashed line that separates baseline data from Intervention data. (E in graph below)

See the graph below for an illustration of the graphing terms.

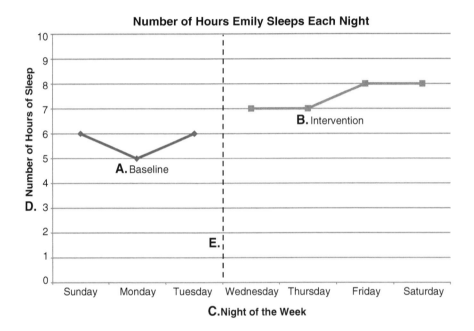

Directions for Graphing by Hand

Emily's parents began implementing an intervention to increase the amount of food Emily consumes. To evaluate the effectiveness of their intervention, Emily's parents have counted the number of bites of food Emily eats each night at dinner for the past week.

This included 3 days before they actually implemented the intervention (the baseline) and 5 points once they started implementing the intervention (progress monitoring). The next step is to graph this data.

Baseline data			Intervention data				
Friday	Saturday	Sunday	Monday	Tuesday	Wednesday	Thursday	Friday
4	4	4	4	7	6	8	9

Step 1: See Appendix D. This is the type of graph on which data can be plotted.

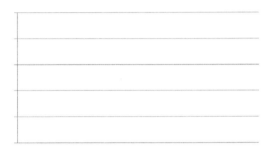

Step 2: Label the horizontal X-axis with the days of the week.

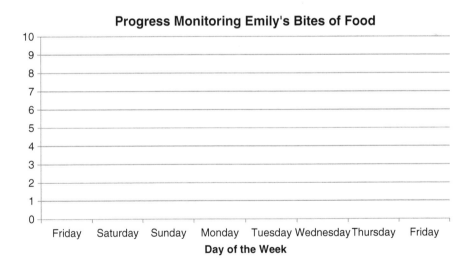

Step 3: Label the vertical *Y*-axis with the behavior and ensure that the scale is appropriate for that behavior (e.g., consider whether or not the scale begins at zero and goes up to or beyond the maximum number of behaviors expected).

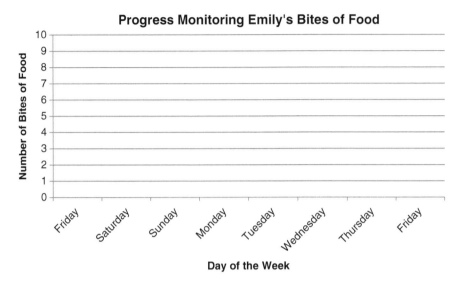

Step 4: Plot the data provided above. Be sure not to connect Baseline and Intervention data.

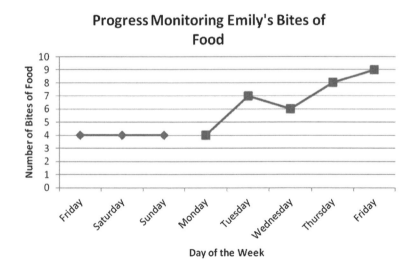

Step 5: Draw a vertical, dotted line between the Baseline and Intervention data to separate them. Then label each.

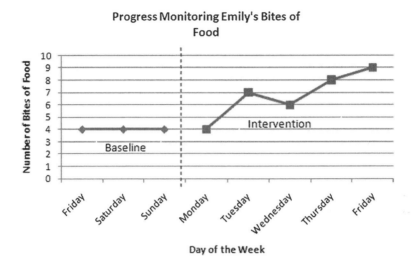

All finished! Now you have a graph of your data.

Computer Graphing

Microsoft Excel is one example of a computer program that makes graphing easy and produces professional-looking graphs. Some people may initially find Excel to be overwhelming, but once you get the hang of it, graphing with Excel is much easier (and more professional looking) than graphing by hand. Included in this text are instructions for graphing with Excel 2007 and Excel 2011.

Graphing with Excel 2007

1. Enter your data in columns as shown below. In column A, enter when the data was collected. This will be your *X*-Axis. In Column B, enter your baseline data for the days you collected it. In Column C, enter your intervention data.

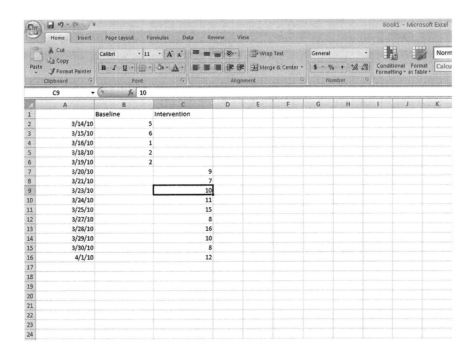

2. Highlight the data by left-clicking on the top left cell, and dragging down and to the right, until all the data are highlighted. Click on the Insert tab, and then click on "Line" in the Charts subsection. Select the "Line with markers" option, which is the first option in the second row.

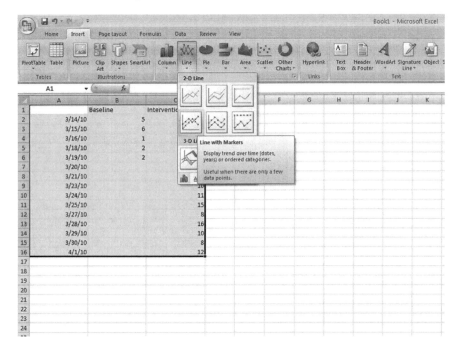

3. You should now have a graph that looks like this one. You will notice a new trio of tabs that appears at the top of the window on the right, colored light green and categorized as Chart Tools, which we will use to modify your graph.

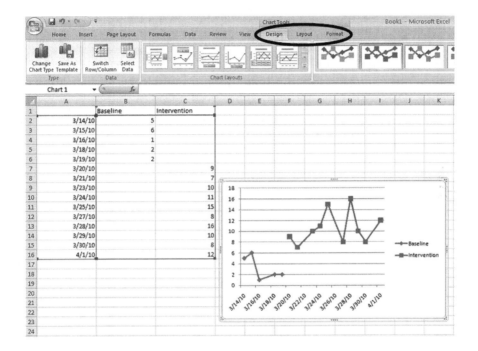

4. Now let's format the axes titles. We will do the *X*-axis title first. Select the
"Layout" tab (in Chart Tools) and click the "Axis Titles" submenu. Select "Title
Below Axis" for the *X*-axis title.

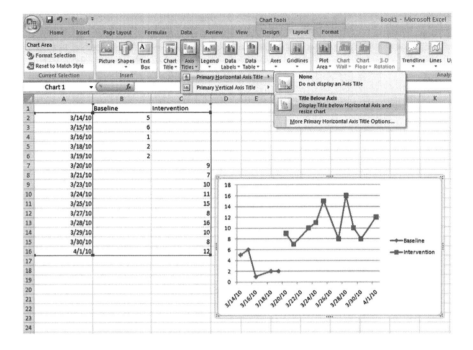

5. Now let's format the Y-axis title. Select the Y-axis from the same "Axis Title" submenu, then click "Rotated Title" to display your title along the Y-axis line. This function will put the Y-axis title along the vertical bar of the graph.

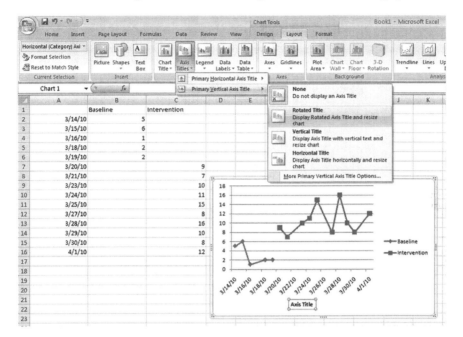

6. Click on the "Axis Title" boxes to enter the desired titles for the X and Y axes.

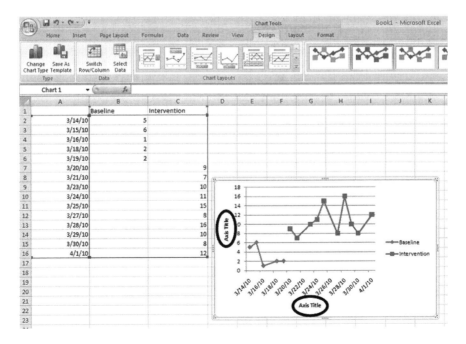

7. The final label on the graph will be the title. Under the "Layout" tab (within
   Chart Tools), select "Chart Title" and select the placement of the Title for the
   graph. The title can then be filled in by clicking on the Chart Title box in the
   graph.

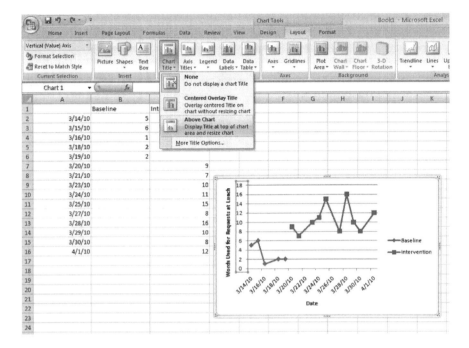

8. Notice that the maximum *Y*-axis value is 18. However, if our goal or aim will exceed 18, we need to extend the scale. We can do this by right-clicking on the *Y*-axis itself. This will bring up a menu with the option "Format Axis."

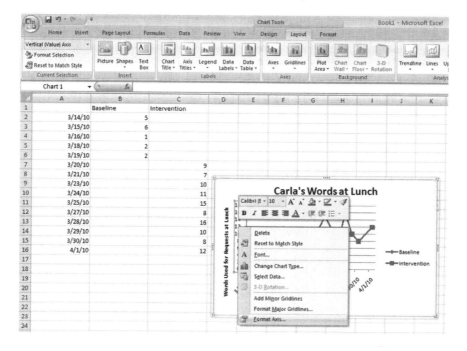

9. In the "Format Axis" toolbox, change Maximum from "Auto" to "Fixed" and
   make the maximum value 30.0. Click "Close."

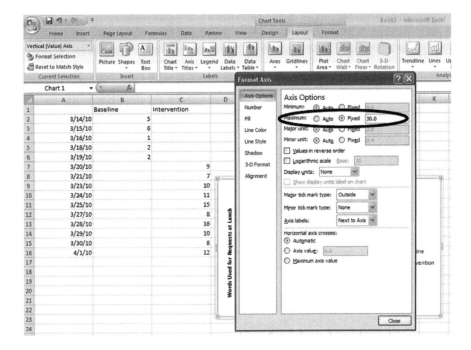

10. Now, right-click within the graph sub-window, but OUTSIDE of the data point area. This will bring up a slightly different window, within which you will see the option "Move Chart."

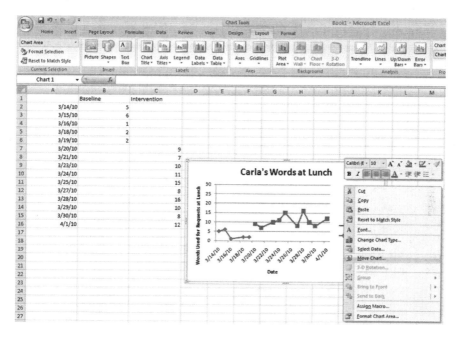

11. In the "Move Chart" window, select the option "New sheet" and type the title
     of your graph. Now click OK.

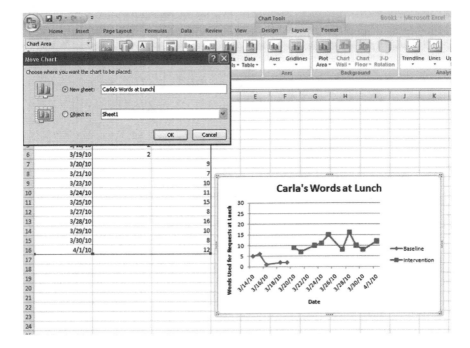

12. Your graph should now look like the one below. You can access the data you typed in before by clicking on "Sheet 1" at the bottom left of the Excel window.

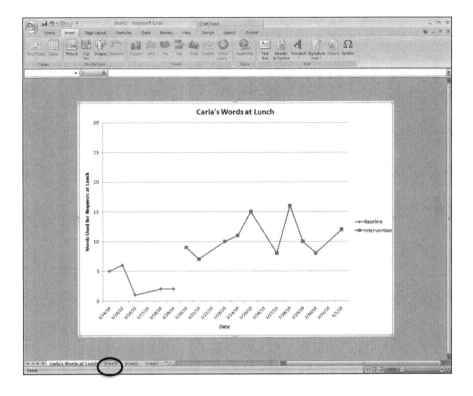

13. Now we are going to add the phase change line to separate the Baseline from
    the Intervention data. Under the Insert tab, select Shapes, and pick the first line
    shown under the Lines submenu.

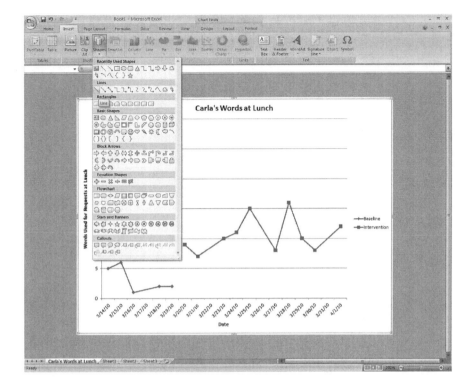

14. You will notice that your pointer has changed into a small cross-hair. Move this new pointer to a point that is between the Baseline and Intervention data. Now, hold down the Shift key on your keyboard, then left-click and drag the pointer vertically downward to the *X*-axis. Release the mouse button and *then* the SHIFT key. (Holding the Shift key keeps the line straight.)

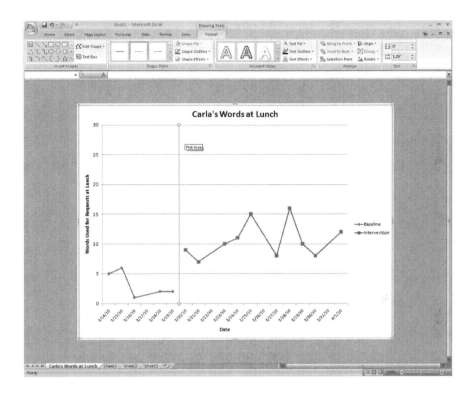

Graphing with Excel 2011

1. Enter your data in columns as shown below. In column A, enter when the data was collected. This will be the *X*-axis. In column B, enter your baseline data for the days you collected it. In column C, enter the data collected while the intervention was in place.

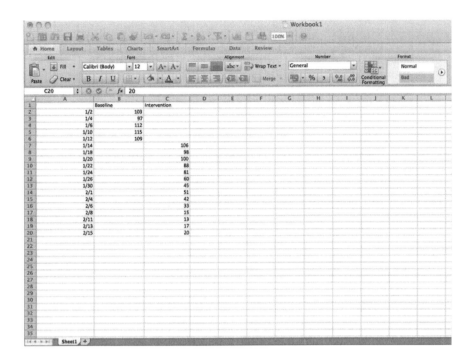

2. Highlight all the information by clicking on the top left cell and holding the mouse while dragging to the bottom right. Make sure all the data are highlighted. Then click on the "Charts" tab at the top and select "Line." The preferred form of Line graph to use is the "Marked Line."

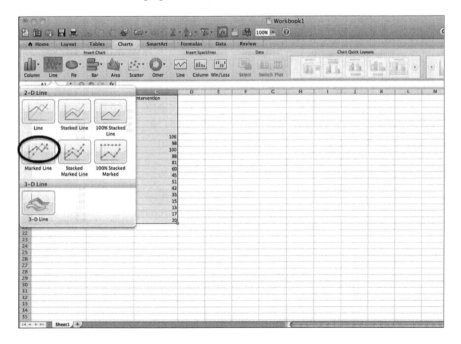

3. Excel will generate a graph to the right of your data. There are also two new tabs: "Chart Layout" and "Format" which contain many functions to changes your graph.

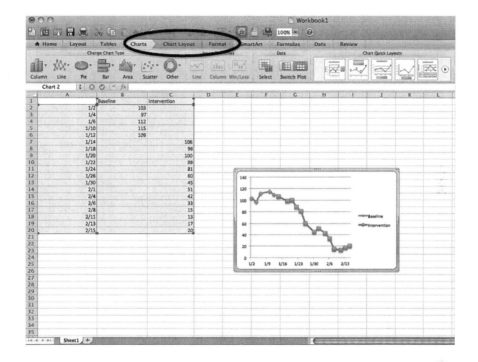

4. The next step is to label your graph so other people can understand what the data represent. First click on the "Chart Layout" tab and then on "Axis Titles." Select the "Horizontal Axis" option and then "Title Below Axis." This will make a text box appear that will allow you to label the graph with the word "Date" in Step 6.

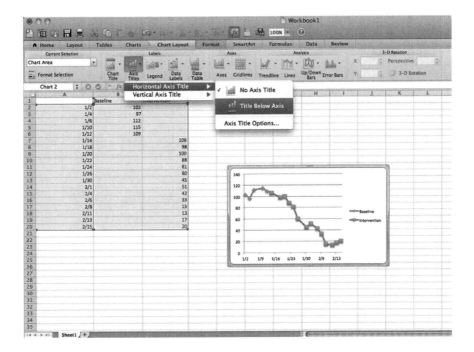

5. Next is the *Y*-axis title. Click "Axis Titles" again but select "Vertical Axis Title" and then select "Rotated Title." A second text box will appear along your *Y*-axis. You will fill this in on the next step.

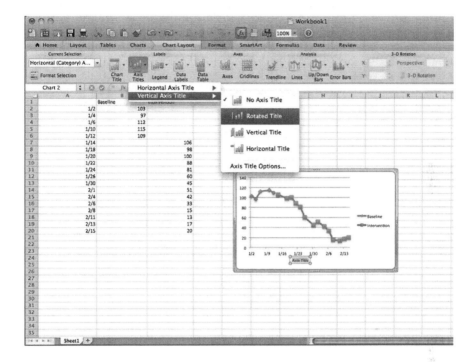

6. Click on both "Axis Title" boxes and enter the desired titles for the X and Y axes. For this graph, the X-axis will get the word "Date" and the Y-axis will be labeled with "Minutes Tantrumming."

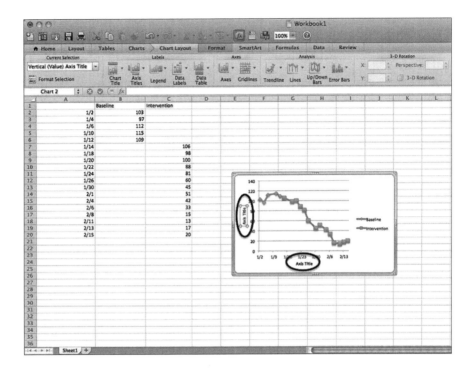

7. The final label on the graph will be the title. Under the "Chart Layout" tab, select "Chart Title" and then click on "Title Above Chart." This will create the final text box or you to type in the title for this graph. In the example below, the graph will be called "Jacob's Tantrums Length."

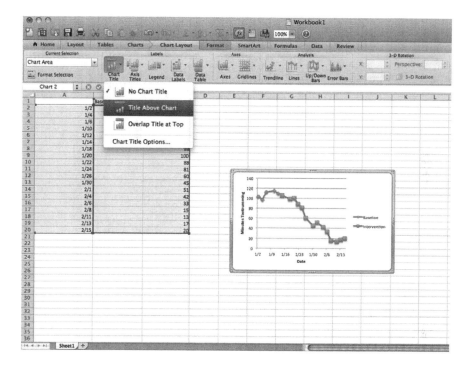

8. Notice that the *Y*-axis goes up to 140 min, but our highest value is 115. To make the graph fit the data better, the *Y*-axis has to be rescaled. To do this, right click when the mouse is over the *Y*-axis. Mac users can hold the "control" button and click the mouse to do this. In the pop-up box that appears, select "Format Axis."

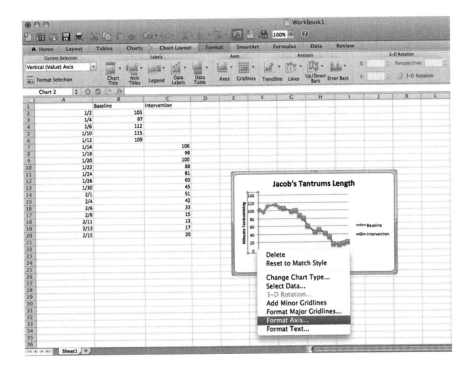

9. In the Format Axis box that pops up, select "Scale" and then change the "Maximum" to reflect the value you want for the top portion of the *Y*-axis. Then select "OK." For this graph, the maximum value will be 120.

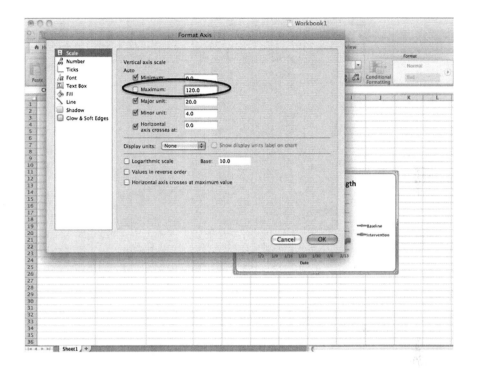

10. Now the graph will be moved so that it can be examined in more detail. To do this, right click on any area outside of the graph lines. A good place is the white space over the "Baseline" word in the Legend. Clicking here will bring up a new menu window where you can select "Move Chart."

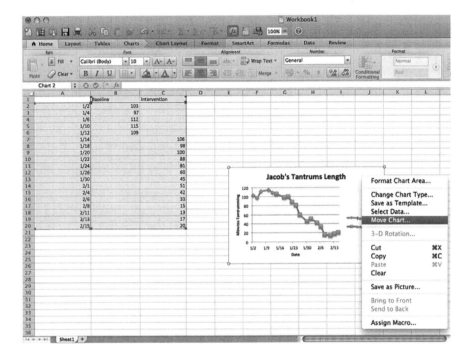

11. Clicking on "Move Chart" opens a new box. Select "New sheet" and then type in the name of your graph. Then click "OK."

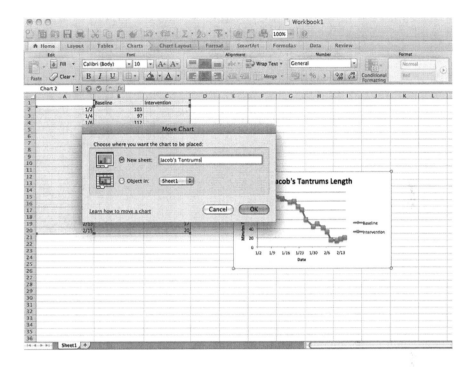

12. You will get a graph on a new sheet. It should look like the one below. You can access the data you typed in before by clicking on "Sheet 1" at the bottom left of the Excel window.

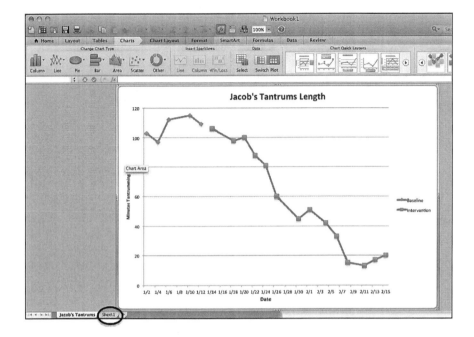

13. The last element to add is the phase change line to separate the Baseline and Intervention phases. At the top of the screen, select "Insert" (between View and Format) and highlight the word "Picture." In the new menu that opened, click on "Shape." This will open a new window with options for shapes.

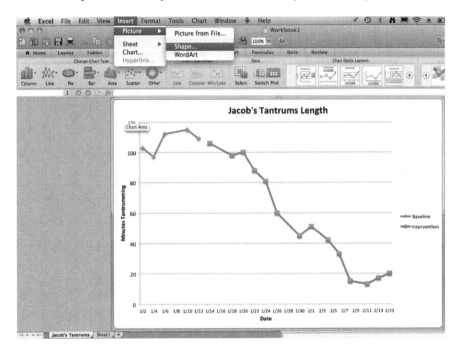

14. In the new window, select "Lines and Connectors." This will bring up several options of lines you can choose from to make your Phase Change Line.

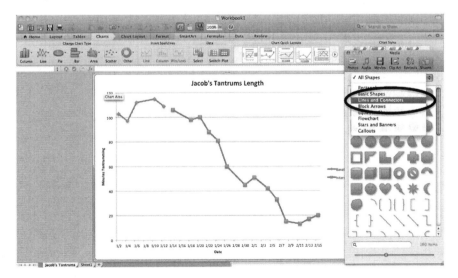

15. After selecting a straight line, you will notice that your cursor has changed into a small cross-hair. Move the cross-hair to a point on the *X*-axis that is between the Baseline and Intervention data. Hold down the "Shift" key on the key board, click your mouse, and drag the mouse upward. When you reach the top of your graph, let go of the mouse and *then* the "Shift" key. Holding down the "Shift" key while dragging keeps the line straight.

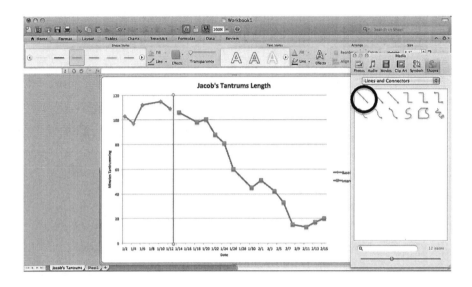

Following these steps will produce a basic graph in Excel. All versions of Microsoft Excel have many features, allowing a user to change the colors of lines, the shape of markers on a line, adding trendlines, etc. The best way to learn about additional functions in Excel is to explore. When you have time, click into different areas and try different features. There is no need to worry about messing up your graph. If something happens to your graph that you did not want to happen, click "Undo" and then keep trying. Just be sure to save you work often as you are going.

Guidelines for Evaluating Outcomes

Once you have five or more progress monitoring data points graphed, you can use your graph to begin evaluating how well your intervention is working. One of three different decisions can be made: (1) continue the intervention; (2) modify the intervention; or (3) discontinue the intervention.

Continue the Intervention

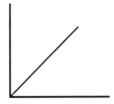

Interventions should continue when they are working, meaning that the desired behavior is increasing (and the challenging behavior is decreasing). When this is the case, the trend of your graph may look like the one above (when graphing the desired behavior). In this situation, continue implementing your intervention.

Modify the Intervention

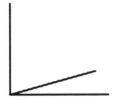

Interventions should be modified when they are working but are working too slowly. Although some interventions work, they may not be working as fast as we would like. Therefore, the intensity of the intervention should be increased, such as increasing the amount of time spent on the intervention.

Discontinue the Intervention

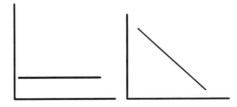

Interventions that have no effect or are detrimental should be discontinued. These progress monitoring lines will have a negative slope or no change at all. In this situation, you should go back to the problem solving process and revise your intervention.

Evaluating Outcomes Examples

Below are four different examples of graphed progress monitoring data and the decisions made about each. Keep in mind that the goal of this intervention was to increase the number of bites of food Emily eats to nine. Ideally, the *progress monitoring* line should increase above zero.

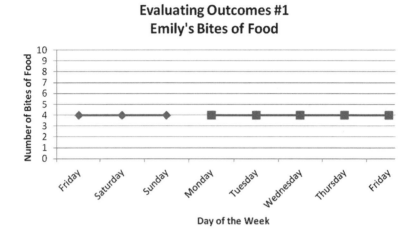

The progress monitoring line is completely flat. This flat line, or slope of zero, indicates that the number of bites of food Emily is eating is not changing and thus not increasing toward the goal of nine bites. Therefore, it appears that this *intervention is not working*. The intervention should be discontinued and a new one should be developed by recycling through the problem solving process. You may also want to check to make sure that the intervention is actually being implemented.

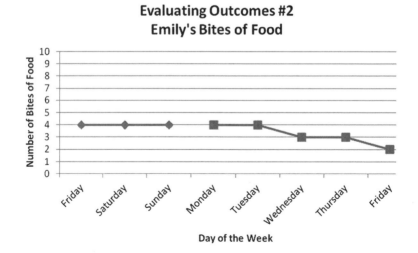

The progress monitoring line on this graph has a negative slope and is moving *toward* zero, meaning that the number of bites of food Emily is eating is decreasing. This line indicates that the intervention is having a detrimental impact on Emily's behavior and *the intervention is not working*. This intervention should be discontinued and a new one should be developed.

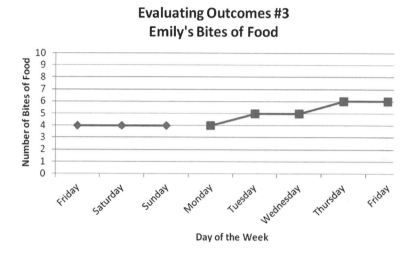

Evaluating Outcomes #3
Emily's Bites of Food

This progress monitoring line has a positive slope and is slowly moving *away* from zero, meaning that the number of bites is increasing toward the goal of nine bites, but slowly. *This intervention is working, but not as quickly as we would like.* This intervention should be adjusted to increase the intensity of the intervention.

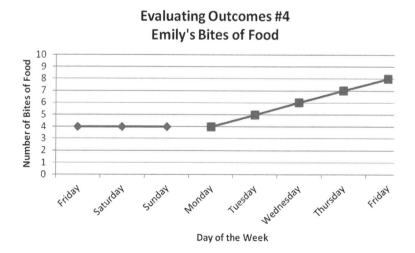

Evaluating Outcomes #4
Emily's Bites of Food

This progress monitoring line has a positive slope and is moving *away* from zero, meaning that the number of bites is increasing toward the goal of nine bites. *This intervention is working*. The intervention should continue as should progress monitoring.

Conclusions

Progress monitoring data makes it possible to determine whether or not the intervention is successful, and can be used to make decisions about the intervention. Graphing data provides a visual display which aids in answering questions as to whether the intervention is working or not, and if it is working as efficiently as intended. Graphs can be completed manually or by using programs such as Microsoft Excel.

Assess Your Knowledge

Use the questions below to assess your knowledge of the information presented in this chapter. Answers appear after the last question.

1. A child is referred to you for frequent head banging. On which axis would you plot head banging?

   a. X-axis
   b. Y-axis
   c. XY-axis
   d. Not enough information to tell

2. What is the primary purpose of collecting baseline data?

   a. To put it on your graph
   b. To be able to tell if your intervention was effective
   c. To show what data you are collecting
   d. To speed up when you can implement your intervention

3. When drawing a graph in Excel, which step comes first?

   a. Label your phases
   b. Format the X-axis
   c. Enter the raw data in columns
   d. Draw the phase change line

4. What is the purpose of the phase change line?

   a. To separate the baseline and intervention data
   b. To show the child's progress during baseline

     c. To show the child's progress during the intervention phase

     d. To label your graph

5. If your graph looks like the graph below, what should be your next step?

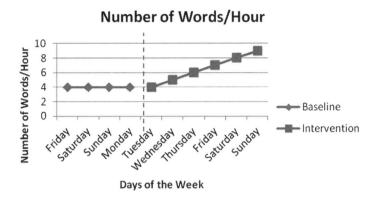

     a. Continue your intervention

     b. Stop the intervention

     c. Change the intervention

     d. Start over with the intervention

6. Data are collected on the number of nights where the child has remained dry through the night (for toileting). On which axis should you place the days of the week?

     a. *X*-axis

     b. *Y*-axis

     c. *XY*-axis

     d. Not enough information to tell

7. If your graph looks like the graph below, what should be your next step?

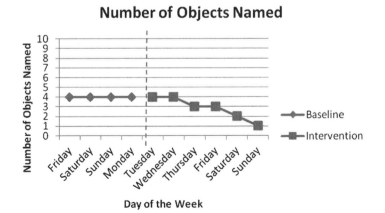

    a. Continue your intervention
    b. Stop the intervention
    c. Change the intervention
    d. Start over with the intervention

8. What is the last step in graphing with Excel?

    a. Label your x- and y-axes
    b. Create the scale for your data
    c. Enter your data in the spreadsheet
    d. Inserting the phase change line.

9. When graphing by hand, which points are not connected?

    a. The baseline points
    b. The last baseline and first intervention data points
    c. The intervention points

10. You are implementing an intervention to increase the number of words a 26-month-old child is saying per hour. Your baseline data shows that the child is saying approximately 1 word per hour. You implement an intervention and track the child's progress. Immediately following the intervention, the child begins using 5 words per hour, and then 10 the next day, and so on. What should you do next?

    a. Continue with the intervention
    b. Modify the intervention
    c. Discontinue the intervention
    d. Change the intervention

Assess Your Knowledge Answers
1) b 2) b 3) c 4) a 5) a 6) a 7) b 8) d 9) b 10) a

Chapter 10
Summary and Conclusions of Best Practices in Providing Services for YCCB

Abstract This final chapter utilizes case studies within the prevention framework in an effort to integrate theories of development, evidence-based practice, behavioral principles, progress monitoring data, and evaluation of outcomes. When possible, the outcomes from each case study are graphically presented so that progress can be observed.

Keywords Evidence-based approaches • Primary, secondary, and tertiary prevention • FBA

Challenging behavior problems are common among young children, and can be transitory, episodic, or chronic. When their families are stressed due to issues such as poverty, disabilities, health or mental health issues, children are at increased risk for more serious behavior problems and subsequently, poor developmental outcomes. Early identification and early intervention are critical approaches to ensuring that all children reach their full potential, leading to happy, healthy, and productive lives.

There are a number of evidence-based approaches available that can help children and their families by educating parents, improving early relationships, and promoting children's social and emotional competence. These approaches are rigorously tested strategies in which research has documented decreases in mental, emotional, and behavioral health problems, and increases in success in the home, school, and community. This manual aims to guide the practitioner in selecting, implementing, and documenting preventive interventions that contribute to healthy development and improved functioning, especially for children who are at increased risk for poor outcomes due to developmental delays and disabilities or environmental factors.

Prevention and early intervention are keys to improving health and well-being of children and their families. Effective prevention/intervention can best be understood within a developmental framework, which is tailored to address the needs of the individual child and their family. Prevention/intervention is a model in which some supports are made available for all children and families in order to maximize development, while more intensive and individualized supports are used to prevent a problem from getting worse or stop a related problem from developing. For example, all children thrive when their parents are nurturing, attentive, and provide consistent discipline, which in turn promotes children's cooperation, motivation, and readiness for school. Many of the challenging behavior problems commonly seen in young children will quickly improve when parents learn to ignore minor misbehavior, and reinforce cooperative behavior, by simply providing praise which is specific, enthusiastic, and immediate. However, some children, especially those challenged with multiple risk factors such as developmental delays, poverty, and insecure attachments will need more intensive interventions in which their families are strengthened and skills are reinforced which improve developmental outcomes.

Prevention and early intervention efforts which incorporate the principles of behavioral theory offer the most evidence for improving children's functioning, and decreasing maladaptive behavior, and have been outlined in this guide. The principles of behavior theory are well defined, and have been supported by thousands of scientific investigations that have helped us to understand how children learn, and what will be most influential towards improving their behavior and teaching new skills. Teaching children social and emotional skills and teaching parents parenting skills decreases problem behaviors and leads to success and achievement. The problem-solving model offers practitioners a practical approach towards understanding the problem behavior, developing, implementing and documenting interventions which will improve functioning, and thereby, healthier developmental outcomes. Ideally, these interventions should take place where children live, play, and learn, and must incorporate their caregivers and family members. Approaches should be developmentally appropriate, culturally sensitive, family centered, and optimistic, if they are to endure.

The following case studies are illustrations of the problem-solving process as it can be applied in early intervention situations. All cases are fictitious, but come from the experiences of the authors in their work with children and families.

Daniel: An Example of Primary Prevention

Daniel and his mother Nicole presented for his regularly scheduled Well-Child Visit. Daniel is 24 months old and Nicole has some concerns regarding his development, specifically:

- He shows no interest in toilet training.
- He seems clumsy and falls when he runs.
- He only uses short phrases (2–3 words) to communicate, which concerns Nicole as Daniel's older sister was talking "up a storm" at this age, and his playgroup friends are more verbal.

With this information the practitioner begins the problem-solving process, and asks Nicole additional questions about her concerns, for example, phrases he might use for requests. She also observes Daniel at play, and observes him as he runs down the hallway. She also asks Nicole to complete the *Ages & Stages Questionnaire* (ASQ; Bricker & Squires, 1999) to document developmental skills. This screening tool is reliable, easy to use, and increases the likelihood that children needing early intervention will be identified (Hamilton, 2006).

Based upon the information gathered through this process, it is determined that Daniel is on target developmentally. Nicole is shown a graph showing Daniel's milestones with those of similar age peers. She is assured that Daniel is meeting expectations, and provided with guidance to help Daniel build his vocabulary. For example, Nicole might describe what is happening during everyday activities, label objects, repeat and extend what Daniel says, sing songs, and read books aloud to him. She is encouraged to put toilet training on hold, until he shows more interest in the process. To help with coordination, she will enroll Daniel in a toddler gymnastics class, where he will have the added benefit of meeting other children his age.

Since Daniel shows no evidence of developmental delays, there is no need for any further assessment. However, Nicole is encouraged to talk to her pediatrician at the next Well-Child Visit if she continues to have concerns. She is provided with handouts about developmental milestones and ideas that turn everyday activities into learning adventures.

Diane: An Example of Secondary Prevention

Diane is a 28-month-old girl who was removed from her parents' home about 5 months ago, due to neglect. Her aunt and uncle are now taking care of her, and are concerned with her temper tantrums. Tantrum behaviors include hitting, crying, and screaming at an ear-piercing level, and last upwards of an hour. She is very resistant to efforts to comfort her.

The Battelle Developmental Inventory Screening Test (BDIST; Newborg, 2005) is used to screen for developmental delays and does not identify concerns which would warrant full assessment for early intervention. However, her caregivers indicate that even though they want to help Diane, they cannot manage her behavior, and are considering returning Diane to foster care because her behavior problems are so problematic.

The practitioner continues the problem-solving process by gathering additional information about Diane's current behavior, including her aunt & uncle's reactions and discipline strategies that they have put into place. The practitioner also gets more information about why Diane was removed from her biological parents' custody, and several important facts emerge. For example, she learned that when Diane's aunt and uncle began taking care of her, she was very underweight, could not feed herself, and was listless. Secondly, Diane's aunt and uncle had little preparation to adapt their lives to that of a young child, had never had children of their own, and they relied on more punitive measures for discipline such as spanking or time out.

In thinking about attachment and how that plays a role in the development of young children, the practitioner hypothesizes that Diane has not had an opportunity to form a secure attachment with adults, and Diane's aunt and uncle do not have knowledge of child development and caregiving skills that will be necessary to help her feel safe and secure.

Diane's caregivers are encouraged to enroll in the local HOT DOCS parenting classes that are held in the community center, so that they will learn more about child development, and meet other parents. In the interim, the practitioner begins working with them on strategies to build a trusting relationship with Diane. The practitioner selects strategies from PCIT as the intervention approach, specifically child directed interaction or CDI. They are directed to spend 5 min every day playing with Diane, during which time they will focus on their use of labeled praise, descriptions of her behavior, and reflection of her words. The practitioner models these skills, and then coaches the caregivers in the implementation. The practitioner is careful to provide ample praise for the caregivers as they practice to enhance their development of these important skills. Diane's aunt and uncle attend all the HOT DOCS classes and begin to utilize the problem-solving chart to help them understand what situations trigger Diane's tantrums, and how they respond to problem behavior. They begin to put prevention efforts in place, such as keeping to predictable routines throughout the day, and giving her warnings prior to transitions.

To monitor changes in Diane's problem behavior, the caregivers kept a record of the number of tantrums per day, which were summarized on a graph. They agreed upon a goal of reducing tantrums to once per day. The data summarize below show that tantrums decreased as caregivers' knowledge and skills improved.

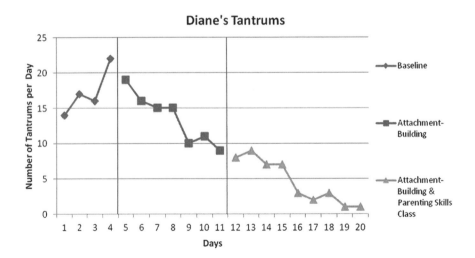

Review of Diane's Case

Although Diane was not experiencing any delays in her development (meeting all milestones), her caregivers clearly needed more assistance in learning how to manage her behavior. By intervening at this point, Diane's behavior was kept from escalating to a point where extensive intervention resources would be needed to address it. Also, the use of a locally available, group parent training program freed up the practitioner's time to work on other concerns (attachment building), and work with other families in need.

Elizabeth: An Example of Tertiary Prevention

Elizabeth, a now 20-month-old girl, was born 8 weeks early, tested positive for cocaine, and spent 2 weeks in the NICU to stabilize her breathing. She was brought home from the hospital by her foster parents, who have since then adopted her. The initial referral concern was that she was not gaining enough weight, showed limited interest in foods, which lead to a diagnosis of failure to thrive. Furthermore, she would not sleep by herself, and became very distressed when people outside of her parents approached her.

The practitioner and parents decided that the first goal they would like to address would be feeding. Elizabeth's current feeding issues included limited acceptance of Stage 2 baby food, gagging or vomiting when given food with textures, and refusal to even hold a spoon. A first step in problem solving was to refer Elizabeth to a gastroenterologist specialist (GI) to make sure that there were no physical issues that would explain her poor feeding, and to a dietician, for recommendations for calorie consumption. No medical problems, including chewing and swallowing, were found that would explain the feeding issues. The GI recommended supplementing Elizabeth's limited food intake with PediaSure for the calories and vitamins.

The practitioner observed Elizabeth during mealtimes and noticed that she would engage in a variety of "resistance" behaviors such as crying, pushing the food away, and sometimes even vomiting. Mealtimes were extended to over 45 minutes, during which time Elizabeth's parents coaxed her to eat, or distracted her with toys, but did not eat themselves. At the conclusion of mealtime, Elizabeth's mother would take her into the family room and hold her in the rocking chair as she consumed a bottle of PediaSure. Based upon these observations, the EIP concluded that Elizabeth's behaviors were escape motivated (for the food), and at the same time, maintained by parents' undivided attention. In addition, she was reinforced with the PediaSure and rocking with her mother after a very unsuccessful mealtime.

A plan was developed to increase Elizabeth's willingness to eat solid foods, which included the following steps: (1) Elizabeth would be offered 5 meals/snacks each day, at consistent times, always in her high chair, and limited to 10 minutes in length (determined by a timer); (2) parents would eat the same food during this time, and communicate their enjoyment; (3) PediaSure would be offered after timer, but Elizabeth had to stay in her chair and drink it by herself; (4) small portions of acceptable food, paired with a new food would be presented; and (5) parents would turn away and ignore all inappropriate mealtime behaviors. Parents and the practitioner developed a social story about eating, which they then read to Elizabeth several times a day.

To document Elizabeth's response to this intervention, The practitioner devoted part of her weekly visit to observing her behaviors during mealtimes, such as touching or tasting new foods, holding her spoon, and swallowing bits of food. Parents were also collecting data on the number of bites of food she consumed.

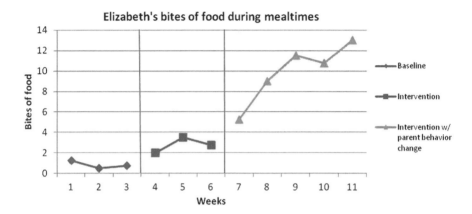

In the first few weeks of implementation, Elizabeth's parents had a difficult time ignoring problem behaviors, and little change was seen in her eating. To assist them, the EIP modeled differential attention, which combines planned ignoring of problem behavior, and attention for any attempt towards independent eating. The practitioner made sure to coach the parents sufficiently so that they were confident in implementing this approach. Within 5 weeks, Elizabeth's feeding problems had greatly improved, and mealtimes became much more enjoyable. Once these gains were solid, her parents indicated a readiness to address sleeping concerns, and along with their EIP problem solved the sleep routine.

Review of Elizabeth's Case

Elizabeth's case falls into the tertiary level of prevention due to the extensive resources needed to change her eating habits and the severity of her problem (resulting in failure to thrive). The problem-solving process had to be revisited several times before an intervention that was effective was developed. In addition, after addressing the most critical issue (feeding), the problem-solving process was applied to Elizabeth's other concerns including sleeping independently.

Easton: An Example of Tertiary Prevention

At 26 months of age, Easton was evaluated for eligibility for Early Steps services due to concerns around speech and language development. He had not met any communication milestones, did not respond to his name, gesture or point. Speech therapy was initiated, however, 6 months later, Easton had still not progressed as well as his mother Karen had hoped. Karen was worried that her son had autism, and wanted a diagnostic evaluation. The practitioner administered the Modified Checklist for Autism in Toddlers (M-CHAT) with Easton's mother to screen Easton for these concerns, and he failed all five critical items. Easton was referred to a pediatric psychologist who completed a comprehensive evaluation and diagnosed Easton with autistic disorder as well as global developmental delays. The team talked with Karen about what this diagnosis might mean for Easton and his future, the types of interventions that are the most beneficial, and asked Karen what she believed were Easton's most pressing needs.

Karen indicated that she really wanted Easton to look at her when she talked with him, and to stop throwing himself on the floor and biting his hand. She also wanted him to be able to play with a toy for more than a few seconds before throwing it aside. These were skills that she believed Easton would need to be successful when he started preschool.

A functional behavior assessment (FBA) was conducted, which included an extensive interview with Karen and observations. The FBA is an example of a problem-solving approach which offers a structured method for identifying the environmental events, circumstances, and interactions which trigger problem behavior, uncover the function of the behaviors, and leads to the development of support strategies to prevent problem behavior and teach new skills. The goal of the FBA is to provide information with respect to intervention strategies that will offer the most benefit to the child. Information gathered from the FBA will lead to the development of a support plan, which includes prevention strategies, techniques for teaching new skills, and changes in responses to any challenging behavior. As with any young child, the intervention strategies work best when they are applied by familiar people, in the home and in other natural settings. As with other problem-solving approaches, reductions in the problem behavior and skill acquisition are monitored and graphed.

The FBA identified that Easton threw himself on the floor and bit his hand when-ever he wanted his mother's attention or when access to a favorite item was restricted. In addition, he engaged in these behaviors whenever he wanted to get out of some-thing, such as cleaning up toys or taking a bath. The support plan included strategies to help Easton gain his mother's attention, to gain access to toys and activities, and to escape undesirable activities. The team decided to teach Easton new skills which would result in gaining his mother's attention, getting a toy or activity, or delaying a transition. Easton was taught to point to a picture showing what he wanted, and his mother or other adults would provide attention or access to the toy or activity. He was also taught to sign "more" when he wanted more time to play before transitioning to a new activity, and it would be allowed for a couple extra minutes. Each time Easton made a request, his mother would repeat the word back to him, using shaping, differential reinforcement, and successive approximations to teach verbal skills.

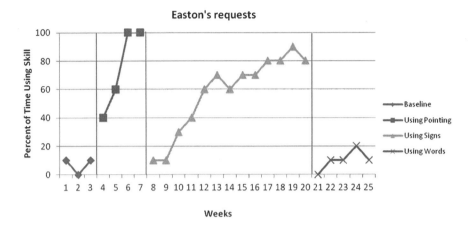

As the data show, Easton progressed well through the first two methods of communication but is still struggling with the use of words. The practitioner might decide to continue teaching the skill for a few more weeks before modifying the intervention to help Easton use words to access his wants and needs.

Notably, many children with autism and as well as with other developmental disabilities need intensive and specific interventions over extended periods of time to develop social and communication skills to prepare them for success in school and other environments. The practitioner has a responsibility to connect families with local resources and help them to plan for their child's transition into the educational system. In the case of Easton, the practitioner helped Karen to find resources and supports in her community, including an integrated primary care setting known as the "medical home," where Easton would have access to health and mental health care. This is especially important for children with diagnosed conditions or who may be at risk for poor outcomes.

Review of Easton's Case

Easton's case represents a tertiary level of services. Easton required very intensive interventions to be able to develop essential skills for the future. Due to Easton's ongoing needs, multiple supports were put in place for Karen and Easton. These supports included enrolling him in a special needs preschool so that he has opportunities to socialize and learn, providing contacts to local autism support groups and resources for Karen, and providing Karen with some extra parenting skills to continue teaching Easton specific behaviors of importance. Throughout the practitioner's work with Easton, interventions were developed based on identified concerns that Karen and the practitioner had for Easton.

Conclusions

Case studies as conceptualized within the prevention framework were used as illustrations of how theories of development, evidence-based practice, and behavioral principles can be integrated in order to make decisions about how much help is needed, and to set individual intervention goals. Data gathered from screening and assessment tools and procedures were used to determine level of support needed, and set treatment goals, while progress monitoring data were used to gauge how well the intervention was working.

Behavioral challenges in young children are common, and most resolve fairly quickly by implementing positive parenting strategies such as routines, positive attention, redirection, and planned ignoring. However, between 9 and 14 % of children have problems serious enough as to require significant assistance (U.S. Department of Health and Human Services, 2010). Providing age appropriate services and supports to these children and their families have proven lifelong benefits, including school completion, less contacts with law enforcement, and ability to live independently.

The prevention model helps to maximize development and saves money by offering parenting and other general information to all families and reserving the more intensive and individualized supports for the most at-risk. By utilizing the problem-solving process, provider teams can determine what help is needed, and determine whether the intervention is working. Evidence-based practice guides providers in selecting scientifically supported interventions that are shown to improve outcomes or reduce complications that might impede healthy development. The most efficacious interventions are founded upon behavioral principles, making knowledge of the science of behavior critical to professionals who work with children and families. Lastly, intervention progress and effectiveness should be documented through data collection and progress monitoring. Graphic representations of these data are easy to make, and show progress towards meeting intervention goals.

Appendix A: Developmental Milestones References

American Academy of Pediatrics, Healthy Children	http://www.healthychildren.org/english/ages-stages/Pages/default.aspx
Center for Disease Control and Prevention, Division of Birth Defects, National Center on Birth Defects and Developmental Disabilities	http://www.cdc.gov/ncbddd/actearly/index.html
3 months	http://www.cdc.gov/ncbddd/actearly/pdf/parents_pdfs/3MonthMilestonesFactShe.pdf
	http://www.healthychildren.org/english/ages-stages/baby/pages/developmental-milestones-3-months.aspx
7 months	http://www.cdc.gov/ncbddd/actearly/pdf/parents_pdfs/7Month.pdf
	http://www.healthychildren.org/English/ages-stages/baby/Pages/Developmental-Milestones-7-Months.aspx
1 year	http://www.cdc.gov/ncbddd/actearly/pdf/parents_pdfs/12MonthMilestonesFactSh.pdf
	http://www.healthychildren.org/English/ages-stages/baby/Pages/Developmental-Milestones-12-Months.aspx
2 years	http://www.cdc.gov/ncbddd/actearly/pdf/parents_pdfs/24MonthMilestonesFactSh.pdf
	http://www.healthychildren.org/English/ages-stages/toddler/Pages/Developmental-Milestones-2-Year-Olds.aspx
3 years	http://www.cdc.gov/ncbddd/actearly/pdf/parents_pdfs/3Year.pdf
	http://www.healthychildren.org/English/ages-stages/preschool/Pages/Developmental-Milestones-3-to-4-Year-Olds.aspx
4 years	http://www.cdc.gov/ncbddd/actearly/pdf/parents_pdfs/4Year.pdf
	http://www.healthychildren.org/English/ages-stages/preschool/Pages/Developmental-Milestones-3-to-4-Year-Olds.aspx
5 years	http://www.cdc.gov/ncbddd/actearly/pdf/parents_pdfs/5Year.pdf
	http://www.healthychildren.org/English/ages-stages/preschool/Pages/Developmental-Milestones-4-to-5-Year-Olds.aspx

K.H. Armstrong et al., *Evidence-Based Interventions for Children with Challenging Behavior*, DOI 10.1007/978-1-4614-7807-2,
© Springer Science+Business Media New York 2014

Appendix B: ABC Chart
for Determining a Behavior's Function

Antecedent	Behavior	Consequence

K.H. Armstrong et al., *Evidence-Based Interventions for Children with Challenging Behavior*, DOI 10.1007/978-1-4614-7807-2,
© Springer Science+Business Media New York 2014

Appendix C: HOT DOCS Behavior Chart

Triggers	Behavior	Consequences
Describe events just before the behavior:	Specifically describe the behavior:	What happened following the behavior?
	Function? To GET or GET OUT OF:	
Preventions	**New Skills**	**New Responses**
What can be done to change or lessen the trigger(s)?	What skills are needed to perform the replacement behavior?	How will others now respond when the new behavior or problem behavior is displayed?

Completed HOT DOCS Chart for Reference*

Triggers	Behavior	Consequences
Describe events just before the behavior:	Specifically describe the behavior:	What happened following the behavior?
• A child is watching T.V. in his room before dinner • He does not respond to a request by his mother to come downstairs • Dad comes into room, turns off T.V. before show ends, and carries child downstairs	Child kicks, screams, cries, throws food off high chair, kicks dinner table, yells "NO!" -these behaviors last for 20 minutes **Function?** To GET or GET OUT OF:	Mom and Dad yell; Dad spanks child; Dad makes child finish food; child is sent back to room as parents argue; child turns on T.V.
Preventions	**New Skills**	**New Responses**
What can be done to change or lessen the trigger(s)?	What skills are needed to perform the replacement behavior?	How will others now respond when the new behavior or problem behavior is displayed?
• Provide warnings/cues that will be soon • Use a visual schedule • Wait for T.V. show to end • Provide choices at dinner (Do you want milk or juice?; red plate or blue plate) • Create a social story for manners at dinner table and prompt expected behaviors	• each appropriate table manners • each communication such as "one more time" • use shaping to develop single tasks related to master skill	For use of new behaviors: • raise • attention • reinforcement For use of problem behavior: • validate feelings • redirect • use Time Out • use a follow-though procedure to ensure compliance

*Adapted from the HOT DOCS Curriculum Manual

K.H. Armstrong et al., *Evidence-Based Interventions for Children with Challenging Behavior*, DOI 10.1007/978-1-4614-7807-2,
© Springer Science+Business Media New York 2014

Appendix D: Graphing by Hand

Graph Name: _____

K.H. Armstrong et al., *Evidence-Based Interventions for Children
with Challenging Behavior*, DOI 10.1007/978-1-4614-7807-2,
© Springer Science+Business Media New York 2014

Glossary

Adaptive behavior A collection of conceptual, social, and practical skills learned by individuals to function in their everyday lives.

Anticipatory guidance Pediatric advice to parents as to what to expect with their infant/child at current and future stages of development.

Attachment theory Highlights the importance of the relationship developed between the parent and child, as well as the detrimental impact on development that results from parental separation, deprivation, or bereavement.

Authoritarian parenting style Described as highly demanding but not responsive parenting. Children tend to be obedient, proficient, but less confident or happy.

Authoritative parenting style Moderately demanding and responsive parenting. Children tend to be happy, capable, and successful.

Baseline data Data collected prior to implementing an intervention.

Cognitive skills Thinking skills, including attention, problem solving, and comprehension.

Cognitive theory Proposes that children progress through a series of developmental stages, in which new information from experiences is taken in (assimilation) and understood based upon their prior understanding and knowledge (accommodation). Piaget believed that children are naturally driven to explore their environment and learn by doing.

Communication skills Ability to get message across to another, through gestures, facial expression, and/or words.

Count The number of times a particular behavior occurs (e.g., the number of words a child says).

Developmental milestone A physical and behavioral sign of maturation that most children demonstrate by a certain age (e.g., responding to own name by 7 months, crawling by 12 months). Developmental milestones are often categorized into one of the following five domains: adaptive, cognitive, communication, motor, and social/emotional.

Differential attention A process involving ignoring of undesirable behavior and attending to the desired behavior to change behavior.

K.H. Armstrong et al., *Evidence-Based Interventions for Children
with Challenging Behavior*, DOI 10.1007/978-1-4614-7807-2,
© Springer Science+Business Media New York 2014

Duration The amount or length of time a behavior occurs (e.g., the number of minutes a tantrum lasts).

Event recording Recording the number of times a behavior occurs over a specific amount of time.

Externalizing behavior A cluster of behaviors expressed outwardly, including aggression, impulsivity, and/or noncompliance.

Extinction Reinforcement of a previously reinforced behavior is discontinued, resulting in decreased in frequency of the behavior in the future.

Frequency/rate The number of occurrences of a behavior within a specific amount of time (e.g., the number of words a child says in an hour).

General Outcome Measurements (GOMs) Similar to a physicians' growth chart, a type of measurement tool that may be used to evaluate progress toward a specific outcome, or long-term desired goal.

Individual Growth and Developmental Indicators (IGDIs) GOMs designed to measure child progress in the areas of adaptive, communication, motor, cognitive, and social/emotional development. Validated tools for infants/toddlers and preschool age children are available.

Internalizing behavior A cluster of behaviors with an inward focus, including behaviors described as anxious, withdrawn, depressed, or lonely.

Interval time sampling methods A type of observation method in which an observer records the presence or absence of a behavior within a specified time interval.

Intervention data Data collected after an intervention is begun.

Intervention implementation Plan which documents *who* will do *what*, *when* it will be done, and *how* long will it be tried.

Intervention integrity The degree to which an intervention is implemented as it was intended, including the frequency and length of sessions and the quality of how the intervention is provided.

Intervention evaluation This step involves revisiting the problem originally identified and examining the data to determine if the intervention is working.

Latency The elapsed between a prompt and a behavioral response (e.g., the number of seconds between an adult saying a child's name and the child looking up).

Learning theory Focuses on the fact that children's behavior is influenced by their experiences with their environment.

Language This is the term used for symbolic communication and includes print, words, sentences, and discourse to express and comprehend unique meanings.

Magnitude The intensity or force with which a behavior is produced (e.g., the volume of a child's voice).

Medical home An approach to providing high quality, comprehensive, and coordinated health care for children in a primary care setting.

Modeling An antecedent stimulus that evokes an imitative behavior. Modeling is a very effective method used to teach children new skills.

Morphology The system of smallest meaningful units of language.

Motor development The acquisition of control or use of large and small muscle masses in the body. This includes perceptual-motor development, and motor coordination, and involves both the brain/central nervous system and muscles.

Narrative recordings An informal observation method that involves recording everything observed.

Partial interval time sampling A type of observation method in which an observer records the behavior when a single instance of the behavior occurs in the interval.

Permissive parenting style Depicted as low demandingness, but highly responsive parenting. Children tend to be self-centered, and do not do well in school.

Phase change line A vertical, dashed line separating data from one phase (i.e., baseline) from another (i.e., intervention).

Pragmatics The system for using language in socially appropriate ways.

Primary prevention Prevention strategies that are intended to promote health and well-being all children and their families. Also may be referred to as Universal Preventions.

Problem analysis In clinical problem solving, refers to developing hypotheses regarding the reason for the problem and identifying interventions that are directly linked to the problem and have a high likelihood of being successful.

Problem identification The first stage of problem solving, in which the problem is clarified, often through history, observations, and screening tools. A discrepancy between a child abilities/skills and where they should fall according to benchmarks or milestones defines the problem.

Progress monitoring The practice of repeated measurements and charting of key skills as a means of determining rates of progress.

Protective factors Refers to characteristics that prevent or make less likely the occurrence of poor outcomes. Sensitive caregivers, supportive relationships, effective schools, safe neighborhoods, and access to health care are key protective factors for children.

Punishment Punishment occurs when a behavior occurs less frequently after a specific response is provided immediately after a behavior. Saying "no", using time out, and spankings are examples of punishment strategies.

Randomized controlled trial A rigorous research design in which an intervention is compared to a control condition (no treatment or other form of therapy) and the participants are randomly assigned to treatments. This type of research design decreases the likelihood that outside factors will significantly impact the results.

Rating scales A type of measurement tool designed to measure a child's behavior based on the report of a caregiver or familiar person. Rating scales typically describe specific behaviors and require a person to answer whether or not a child exhibits that behavior (e.g., "Does the child say 10 or more different words?"). Since the caregiver completes the rating scales by considering past observances of the child's behavior, the child does not need to be present during the administration. Rating scales can be completed independently by the caregiver or through an interview between an examiner and the caregiver.

Reinforcement (positive and negative) Reinforcement increases the likelihood that a behavior will occur in the future. If the behavior is increased following the consequence, the consequence is referred to as positive reinforcement (e.g. praising child for sharing). If the behavior increases when the consequence is stopped or removed, the consequence is referred to as negative reinforcement (turning off vacuum to stop child crying).

Replication study A research study which seeks to confirm findings from a previous study, sometimes with different populations or groups of people.

Risk factors Characteristics that make poor outcomes more likely to occur. Risk factors for early childhood include poverty, parental mental health problems and substance abuse, unsafe neighborhoods, health and developmental problems.

Schedules of reinforcement A rule that establishes the probability that a behavior will produce reinforcement. Continuous reinforcement should be used to strengthen new behaviors, while intermittent reinforcement will maintain behaviors.

Screening The use of a brief measurement tool designed to identify risk for health or developmental problems, and need for referral for more comprehensive assessment. Sensitivity (true positives; 70–80 % are identified) and specificity (true negatives; at least 80 % are identified) are important to consider in selecting screening tools.

Secondary prevention/intervention Intervention strategies which are targeted toward at-risk populations to teach skills and prevent poor outcomes in the future. This is also referred to as Selected Prevention.

Shaping A process in which reinforcement is provided following behaviors that approximate the goal or desired behavior outcome. Shaping is often used to teach children new skills.

Social/emotional development Refers to ability to recognize and regulate emotions, form relationships, and behave as expected in social situations. Social/emotional competence leads to better school achievement, better physical and mental health, and increased happiness.

Subclinical symptoms Having the majority of symptoms of a disorder but not meeting all diagnostic criteria *or* falling just below a clinical score on a rating scale.

Tertiary prevention/intervention These interventions are the most intensive, and are intended for children already experiencing significant difficulties and their families. This is also referred to as Indicated Prevention, as the interventions address current issues and prevent more serious outcomes.

Uninvolved parenting style Parenting style, in which there are few demands, low responsiveness, and little communication. Children are less competent, may have poor self-esteem, and lack self-control.

Well-child visit Refer to regularly scheduled appointments to a pediatrician's office for preventive care, to support healthy growth and development. The American Academy of Pediatrics (AAP, 2006) recommends that pediatricians screen for developmental delays at 9, 18, 24, and 30 months visits. In addition, AAP recommends that an autism specific tool be used at the 18 and 24 months visits.

Whole interval time sampling A type of observation method in which an observer records the behavior only when it is emitted throughout an entire interval.

X-axis The horizontal axis of a graph where time should be indexed.

Y-axis The vertical axis of a graph where the behavior should be indexed.

References

Agazzi, H., Salinas, A., Williams, J., Chiriboga, D., Ortiz, C., & Armstrong, K. (2010). Adaption of a behavioral parent-training curriculum for Hispanic caregivers: HOT DOCS Espanol. *Infant Mental Health Journal, 31*(2), 182–200.

Ainsworth, M. D. S., & Bowlby, J. (1991). An ethological approach to personality development. *American Psychologist, 46*, 331–341.

American Academy of Pediatrics. (1999). *Toilet training guidelines*. Retrieved February 1, 2012, from https://www2.aap.org/sections/scan/practicingsafety/Toolkit_Resources/Module7/toilet_training_clinicians.pdf

American Academy of Pediatrics. (2006). *Developmental surveillance and screening of infants and young children: Clinical practice guidelines*. Retrieved December 1, 2010, from http://www.aap.org/healthtopics/early.cfm

American Psychiatric Association. (2000). *Diagnostic and statistical manual of mental disorders* (Rev. 4th ed.). Washington, DC: Author.

Armstrong, K., Agazzi, H., Childres, J., & Lilly, C. (2012). HOT DOCS: Ayudando a nuestros ninos desarrollando sus habilidades (2da. Edicion-revisada). Tampa, FL: University of South Florida.

Armstrong, K., Hornbeck, M., Beam, B., Mack, K., & Popkave, K. (2006). Evaluation of a curriculum designed for caregivers of young children with challenging behavior. *Journal of Early Childhood and Infant Psychology, 2*, 52–61.

Armstrong, K., Kohler, W., & Lilly, C. (2009). Managing sleep disorders from a to zzz's: A pediatrician's guide to managing sleep problems. *Contemporary Pediatrics, 26*(3), 28–36.

Armstrong, K., Lilly, C., Agazzi, H., & Williams, J. (2010). HOT DOCS: Helping Our Toddlers Developing Our Children's Skills Provider Manual (2nd ed.) Tampa, FL: University of South Florida.

Athanasiou, M. (2007). Review of the Battelle Developmental Inventory (2nd ed.). *In the Seventeenth Mental Measurements Yearbook*. Retrieved from EBSCO Mental Measurements Yearbook database.

Aylward, G. P. (1995). *Bayley Infant Neurodevelopmental Screener*. San Antonio, TX: Pearson Education.

Azrin, N. H., & Foxx, R. M. (1974). *Toilet training in less than a day*. New York: Pocket Books.

Baggett, K., & Carta, J. J. (2006). Using assessment to guide social-emotional intervention for very young children: An individual growth and development indicator (IDI) of parent-child interaction. *Young Exceptional Children Monograph Series, 8*, 67–76.

Bagnato, S. J. (2006). The authentic alternative for assessment in early intervention: An emerging evidence-based practice. *Journal of Early Intervention, 28*, 17–22.

Bagnato, S. J., Neisworth, J. T., & Munson, S. M. (1997). *Linking assessment and early intervention: An authentic curriculum-based approach* (3rd ed.). Baltimore: Brookes.

K.H. Armstrong et al., *Evidence-Based Interventions for Children with Challenging Behavior*, DOI 10.1007/978-1-4614-7807-2,
© Springer Science+Business Media New York 2014

Bagner, D. M., & Eyberg, S. M. (2007). Parent-child interaction therapy for disruptive behavior in children with mental retardation: A randomized controlled trial. *Journal of Clinical Child and Adolescent Psychology, 36*, 418–429.

Bandura, A. (1977). *Social learning theory*. Oxford, England: Prentice Hall.

Barnett, W. S., Jung, K., Yarosz, D. J., Thomas, J., Hornbeck, A., Stechuk, R., et al. (2008). Educational effects of the Tools of the Mind curriculum: A randomized trial. *Early Childhood Research Quarterly, 23*, 299–313.

Baum, C. G., Reyna McGlone, C. L., & Ollendick, T. H. (1986). *The efficacy of behavioral parent training: Behavioral parent training plus clinical self-control training, and a modified STEP program with children referred for noncompliance*. Paper presented at the meeting of the Association for Advancement of Behavior Therapy, Chicago.

Baumrind, D. (1966). Effects of authoritative parental control on child behavior. *Child Development, 37*(4), 887–907.

Baumrind, D. (1967). Child care practices anteceding three patterns of preschool behavior. *Genetic Psychology Monographs, 75*, 43–88.

Baumrind, D. (1991). The influence of parenting style on adolescent competence and substance use. *Journal of Early Adolescence, 11*, 56–95.

Benish, J. K. (2007). Review of the Bayley Scales of Infant and Toddler Development (3rd ed.). *In the Seventeenth Mental Measurements Yearbook*. Retrieved from EBSCO Mental Measurements Yearbook database.

Bischoff, L. (2012). Parents' Evaluation of Developmental Status. *In the Fourteenth Mental Measurements Yearbook*. Retrieved from EBSCO Mental Measurements Yearbook database.

Blum, N. J., Taubman, B., & Nemeth, N. (2003). Relationship between age at initiation of toilet training and duration of training: A prospective study. *Pediatrics, 111*(4), 810–814.

Bondy, A. S., & Frost, L. A. (1994). The picture exchange system. *Focus on Autism and Other Developmental Disabilities, 9*(3), 1–19.

Bor, W., Sanders, M. R., & Markie-Dadds, C. (2002). The effects of the Triple P-Positive Parenting Program on preschool children with co-occurring disruptive behavior and attentional/hyperactive difficulties. *Journal of Abnormal Child Psychology, 30*(6), 571–587.

Bower, P., & Gilbody, S. (2005). Stepped care in psychological therapies: Access, effectiveness, and efficiency. *The British Journal of Psychiatry, 186*, 11–17.

Brauner, C., & Stephens, C. (2006). Estimating prevalence of serious emotional and behavioral disorders: Challenges and recommendations. *Public Health Reports, 121*, 303–310.

Bricker, D., & Squires, J. (2009). *Ages & Stages Questionnaires, ASQ-3: A parent-completed child-monitoring system* (3rd ed.). Baltimore: Brookes.

Bricker, D., & Squires, J. (1999). *Ages and Stages Questionnaires (ASQ): A parent-completed child-monitoring system* (2nd ed.). Baltimore, MD: Paul H. Brookes Publishing Co.

Brigance, A. H., & Glascoe, F. P. (2010). *Brigance Infant and Toddler Screen*. North Billerica, MA: Curriculum Associates.

Briggs-Gowan, M. J., & Carter, A. S. (2006). *Brief Infant Toddler Social Emotional Assessment*. San Antonio, TX: Pearson Education.

Brinkmeyer, M. Y., & Eyberg, S. M. (2003). Parent-child interaction therapy for oppositional children. In A. E. Kazdin & J. R. Weisz (Eds.), *Evidence-based psychotherapies for children and adolescents*. New York: Guilford.

Bronfenbrenner, U. (1979). *The ecology of human development: Experiments by nature and design*. Cambridge, MA: Harvard University Press.

Brown, W. H., Odom, S. L., & Conroy, M. (2001). An intervention hierarchy from promoting preschool children's peer interaction in naturalistic environments. *Topics in Early Childhood Special Education, 21*, 162–175.

Buckhalt, J. A., Wolfson, A., & El-Sheikh, M. (2007). Children's sleep, academic performance, and school behavior. *NASP Communique, 35*, 40–43.

Carey, K. (2012). Review of Communication and Symbolic Behavior Scales Developmental Profile: First Normed Edition. *In the Sixteenth Mental Measurements Yearbook*. Retrieved from EBSCO Mental Measurements Yearbook database.

Carta, J. J., Greenwood, C. R., Luze, G. J., Cline, G., & Kuntz, S. (2004). Developing a general outcome measure of growth in social skills for infants and toddlers. *Journal of Early Intervention, 26*, 91–114.

Carter, A. S., Wagmiller, R. J., Gray, S. A. O., McCarthy, K. J., Horwitz, S. M., & Briggs-Gowan, M. J. (2010). Prevalence of DSM-iv disorder in a representative, healthy birth cohort at school entry: Sociodemographic risks and social adaptation. *Journal of the American Academy of Child and Adolescent Psychiatry, 49*, 686–698.

Center for Disease Control and Prevention. (2011). *Child development.* Retrieved February 12, 2013, from http://www.cdc.gov/NCBDDD/childdevelopment/facts.htm

Chaffin, M., Silovsky, J. F., Funderburk, B., Valle, L. A., Brestan, E. V., Balachova, T., et al. (2004). Parent-child interaction therapy with physically abusive parents: Efficacy for reducing future abuse reports. *Journal of Consulting and Clinical Psychology, 72*, 500–510.

Chambless, D. L., & Hollon, S. D. (1998). Defining empirically supported therapies. *Journal of Consulting and Clinical Psychology, 66*, 7–18.

Chorpita, B. F. (2003). The frontier of evidence-based practice. In A. E. Kazdin & J. R. Weisz (Eds.), *Evidence-based psychotherapies for children and adolescents* (pp. 42–59). New York: Guilford.

Childres, J., Shaffer-Hudkins, E., & Armstrong, K. (in press). *Helping Our Toddlers, Developing Our Children's Skills: A problem-solving approach for parents of young children with autism spectrum disorders.* Journal of Early Childhood and Infant Psychology.

Cohen, J. A., Deblinger, E., Mannarino, A. P., & Steer, R. A. (2004). A multi-site randomized controlled trial for sexually abused children with PTSD symptoms. *Journal of the American Academy of Child and Adolescent Psychiatry, 43*, 393–402.

Cohen, J. A., & Mannarino, A. P. (1996). A treatment outcome study for sexually abused preschool children: Initial findings. *Journal of the American Academy of Child and Adolescent Psychiatry, 35*, 42–50.

Cohen, J. A., & Mannarino, A. P. (1997). A treatment study of sexually abused preschool children: Outcome during a one year follow-up. *Journal of the American Academy of Child and Adolescent Psychiatry, 36*, 1228–1235.

Cohen, J. A., Mannarino, A. P., & Deblinger, E. (2006). *Treating trauma and traumatic grief in children and adolescents.* New York: Guilford.

Cohen, J. A., Mannarino, A. P., & Knudsen, K. (2005). Treating sexually abused children: 1 year follow-up of a randomized controlled trial. *Child Abuse & Neglect, 29*, 135–145.

Coie, J. K., & Dodge, K. A. (1998). Aggression and antisocial behavior. In W. Damon (Editor in Chief) & N. Eisenberg (Vol. Ed.), *Handbook of child psychology* (5th ed., Vol. 3). Social, emotional, and personality development. New York: Wiley.

Coleman, M. R., Buysse, V., & Neitzel, J. (2006). *Recognition and response: An early intervening system for young children at risk for learning disabilities. Full report.* Chapel Hill: The University of North Carolina at Chapel Hill, FPG Child Development Institute.

Connell, S., Sanders, M. R., & Markie-Dadds, C. (1997). Self-directed behavioral family intervention for parents of oppositional children in rural and remote areas. *Behavior Modification, 21*(4), 379–408.

Cooper, J. O., Heron, T. E., & Heward, W. L. (2007). *Applied behavior analysis* (2nd ed.). Upper Saddle River, NJ: Prentice Hall.

Cowen, P. S. (2001). Effectiveness of a parent education intervention for at-risk families. *Journal of the Society of Pediatric Nurses, 6*(2), 73–82.

Curtiss, H., Armstrong, K., & Lilly, C. (2008). Positive behavior support and pediatric feeding problems: A case study. *Journal of Early Childhood and Infant Psychology, 4*, 94–109.

Dadds, M. R., Sanders, M. R., Behrens, B. C., & James, J. E. (1987). Marital discord and child behavior problems: A description of family interactions during treatment. *Journal of Clinical Child Psychology, 16*(3), 192–203.

Dawson, G., Rogers, S., Munson, J., Smith, M., Winter, J., Greenson, J., et al. (2010). Randomized, controlled trial of an intervention for toddlers with autism: The Early Start Denver Model. *Pediatrics, 125*(1), e17–e24.

Deblinger, E., Lippman, J., & Steer, R. (1996). Sexually abused children suffering posttraumatic stress symptoms: Initial treatment outcome findings. *Child Maltreatment, 1*, 310–321.

Devereux Early Childhood Initiative. (2000). Pilot study of the Devereux Early Childhood Assessment Program-Year 1. *Devereux early childhood initiative: Research bulletin #1*. Retrieved from http://www.devereux.org/site/PageServer?pagename=deci_research_bulletins

Diamond, A., Barnett, W. S., Thomas, J., & Munro, S. (2007). Preschool program improves cognitive control. *Science, 318*, 1387–1388.

Dishion, T. J., French, D. C., & Patterson, G. R. (1995). The development and ecology of antisocial behavior. In D. Cicchetti & D. J. Cohen (Eds.), *Developmental psychopathology* (Vol. 2). Oxford, England: Wiley.

Dodge, D. T., & Colker, L. J. (1988). *The creative curriculum*. Washington, DC: Teaching Strategies.

Domitrovich, C. E., Cortes, R. C., & Greenberg, M. T. (2007). Improving young children's social and emotional competence: A randomized trial of the preschool "PATHS" curriculum. *Journal of Primary Prevention, 28*(2), 67–91.

Drotar, D., & Hurwitz, H. M. (2005). *The Cleveland Eastern Suburban Born to Learn Program: Final report*. Cleveland: Case Western University School of Medicine.

Dubas, J. S., Lynch, K. B., Galano, J., Geller, S., & Hunt, D. (1998). Preliminary evaluation of a resiliency-based preschool substance abuse and violence prevention project. *Journal of Drug Education, 28*, 235–255.

Eckenrode, J., Campa, M., Luckey, D. W., Henderson, C. R., Cole, R., Kitzman, H., et al. (2010). Long-term effects of prenatal and infancy nurse home visitation on the life course of youths: 19-year follow-up of a randomized trial. *Archives of Pediatric and Adolescent Medicine, 164*(1), 9–15.

Eckenrode, J., Ganzel, B., Henderson, C. R., Smith, E., Olds, D. L., Powers, J., et al. (2000). Preventing child abuse and neglect with a program of nurse home visitation: The limiting effects of domestic violence. *Journal of the American Medical Association, 284*, 1385–1391.

Elliott, S. N., Roach, A. T., & Beddow, P., III. (2008). Best practices in preschool school skills training. In A. Thomas & J. Grimes (Eds.), *Best practices in school psychology V* (pp. 1531–1546). Bethesda, MD: National Association of School Psychologists.

Epstein, M. H., & Walker, H. M. (2002). Special education: Best practices and First Step to Success. In B. J. Burns & K. Hoagwood (Eds.), *Community treatment for youth: Evidence-based interventions for severe emotional and behavioral disorders* (pp. 179–197). New York: Oxford University Press.

Eyberg, S. M., Nelson, M. M., & Boggs, S. R. (2008). Evidence-based psychosocial treatments for children and adolescents with disruptive behavior. *Journal of Clinical Child and Adolescent Psychology, 37*(1), 215–237.

Feis, C. L., & Simons, C. (1985). Training preschool children in interpersonal problem solving skills: A replication. *Prevention in Human Services, 3*(4), 59–70.

Ferber, R. (2009). *Solve your baby's sleep problems*. New York: Fireside.

Fernandez, M. A., Butler, A., & Eyberg, S. M. (2009). Treatment outcome for African American families in parent-child interaction therapy: A Pilot Study. Manuscript under review.

Fox, L., Carta, J., Strain, P. S., Dunlap, G., & Hemmeter, M. L. (2010). Response to intervention and the pyramid model. *Infants and Young Children, 23*(1), 3–13.

Friedrich, W. N., Fisher, J., Broughton, D., Houston, M., & Shafran, C. R. (1998). Normative sexual behavior in children: A contemporary sample. *Pediatrics, 101*(4), e9.

Garfinkle, A., & Schwartz, I. (2002). Peer imitation: Increasing social interactions in children with autism and other developmental disabilities in inclusive preschool classrooms. *Topics in Early Childhood Special Education, 22*, 26–38.

Glascoe, F. P. (2008). *PEDS: Developmental Milestones (PEDS:DM)*. Nashville, TN: PEDSTest.com.

Glascoe, F. P. (2010). *Parents' Evaluation of Developmental Status (PEDs)*. Nashville, TN: PEDSTest.com.

Golly, A., Sprague, J., Walker, H., Beard, K., & Gorham, G. (2000). The First Step to Success Program: An analysis of outcomes with identical twins across multiple baselines. *Behavioral Disorders, 25*, 170–182.

Golova, N., Alario, A. J., Vivier, P. M., Rodriguez, M., & High, P. C. (1999). Literacy promotion for Hispanic families in a primary care setting: A randomized, controlled trial. *Pediatrics, 103*(5), 993–997.

Gray, C., Dutkiewicz, M., Fleck, C., Moore, L., Cain, S. L., Lindrup, A., et al. (1994). *The social story book.* Arlington TX: Future Horizons.

Greenberg, M. T., & Speltz, M. (1991). Emotion regulation, self control, and psychopathology. In C. A. Kusché, D. Cicchetti, & S. Toth (Eds.), *Internalizing and externalizing expressions of dysfunction. Rochester Symposium on Developmental Psychopathology* (Vol. 2, pp. 21–55). Hillsdale, NJ: Lawrence Erlbaum Associates, Inc.

Greenwood, C. R., Carta, J. J., Walker, D., Hughes, K., & Weathers, M. (2006). Preliminary investigations of the application of the Early Communication Indicator (ECI) for infants and toddlers. *Journal of Early Intervention, 28,* 178–196.

Greenwood, C. R., Luze, G. J., Cline, G., Kuntz, S., & Leitschuh, C. (2002). Developing a general outcome measure of growth in movement for infants and toddlers. *Topics in Early Childhood Special Education, 22,* 143–157.

Greenwood, C. R., Walker, D., Carta, J.J., & Higgins, S. (2006). Developing a general outcome measure of growth in the cognitive abilities of children 1 to 4 years old: The Early Problem-Solving Indicator. *School Psychology Review, 35*(4), 535–551.

Gross, D., Fogg, L., Webster-Stratton, C., Garvey, C., Julion, W., & Grady, J. (2003). Parent-training of toddlers in day care in low-income urban communities. *Journal of Consulting and Clinical Psychology, 71*(2), 261–278.

Guzell, J., & Vernon-Feagans, L. (2004). Parental perceived control over caregiving and its relationship to parent-infant interaction. *Child Development, 75*(1), 134–146.

Hair, E. C., & Graziano, W. G. (2003). Self-esteem, personality and achievement in high school: A prospective longitudinal study in Texas. *Journal of Personality, 71*(6), 971–994.

Hamilton, S. (2006). Screening for developmental delay: Reliable, easy to use tools. *Journal of Family Practice, 55*(5), 1–9.

Hanf, C. (1969). *A two-stage program for modifying maternal controlling during mother-child interaction.* Paper presented at the meeting of the Western Psychological Association, Vancouver, BC, Canada.

Hanf, C. (1970). Shaping mothers to shape their children's behavior. Unpublished manuscript, University of Oregon Medical School.

Hanig, K. (2012). Review of ages & stages questionnaires: A parent-completed, child-monitoring system (3rd ed.). *In the Eighteenth Mental Measurements Yearbook.* Retrieved from EBSCO Mental Measurements Yearbook database.

Hickson, G. B., Altemeier, W. A., & O'Connor, S. (1983). Concerns of mothers seeking care in private pediatric offices: Opportunities for expanding services. *Pediatrics, 72,* 619–624.

High, P., Hopman, M., LaGasse, L., & Linn, H. (1998). Evaluation of a clinic-based program to promote book sharing and bedtime routines among low-income urban families with young children. *Archives of Pediatrics & Adolescent Medicine, 152,* 459–465.

High, P., LaGasse, L., Becker, S., Ahlgren, I., & Gardner, A. (2000). Literacy promotion in primary care pediatrics: Can we make a difference? *Pediatrics, 105*(4), 927–934.

Horn, E. M. (2003). Assessment, Evaluation, and Programming System for Infants and Children, Second Edition. (Book Review). *Topics in Early Childhood Special Education, 23*(1), 41–42.

Hoyson, M., Jamieson, B., & Strain, P. S. (1984). Individualized and group instruction of normally developing and autistic-like children: The LEAP curriculum model. *Journal of the Division for Early Childhood, 8,* 157–172.

Ikeda, M., Neessen, E., & Witt, J. (2008). Best practices in universal screening. In A. Thomas & J. Grimes (Eds.), *Best practices in school psychology V* (pp. 103–114). Washington, DC: National Association of School Psychologists.

Ireland, J. L., Sanders, M. R., & Markie-Dadds, C. (2003). The impact of parent training on marital functioning: A comparison of two group versions of the Triple P-Positive Parenting Program for parents of children with early-onset conduct problems. *Behavioural and Cognitive Psychotherapy, 31,* 127–142.

Jenkins, S., Bax, M., & Hart, H. (1980). Behaviour problems in pre-school children. *Journal of Child Psychology and Psychiatry, 21*(1), 5–17.

Joanna Briggs Institute. (2004). The effectiveness of interventions for infant colic. *Best Practice, 8*(2), 1–6.

Kazak, A. E. (2006). Pediatric Psychosocial Preventative Health Model (PPPHM): Research, practice and collaboration in pediatric family systems medicine. *Families, Systems & Health, 24*, 381–395.

Kellogg, N. D. (2009). Clinical report: The evaluation of sexual behaviors in children. *Pediatrics, 124*(3), 992–998.

Kitzman, H., Olds, D. L., Cole, R. E., Hanks, C. A., Anson, E. A., Arcoleo, K. J., et al. (2010). Enduring effects of prenatal and infancy home visiting by nurses on children. *Archives of Pediatric and Adolescent Medicine, 164*(5), 412–418.

Kitzman, H., Olds, D. L., Henderson, C. R., Hanks, C., Cole, R., Tatlebaum, R., et al. (1997). Effect of prenatal and infancy home visitation by nurses on pregnancy outcomes, childhood injuries, and repeated childbearing: A randomized controlled trial. *Journal of the American Medical Association, 278*(8), 644–652.

Kitzman, H., Olds, D. L., Sidora, K., Henderson, C. R., Hanks, C., Cole, R., et al. (2000). Enduring effects of nurse home visitation on maternal life course: A three-year follow-up of a randomized trial. *Journal of the American Medical Association, 283*, 1983–1989.

Komro, K., Flay, B., & Biglan, A. (2011). Creating nurturing environments: A science-based framework for promoting child health and development within high-poverty neighborhoods. *Clinical Child and Family Psychology Review, 14*, 111–134.

Konold, T. R. (2007). Review of ITSEA/BITSEA: Infant-Toddler and Brief Infant-Toddler Social and Emotional Assessment. *In the Seventeenth Mental Measurements Yearbook*. Retrieved from EBSCO Mental Measurements Yearbook database.

Konold, T. R., & Pianta, R. C. (2005). Empirically-derived, personoriented patterns of school readiness in typically-developing children: Description and prediction to first-grade achievement. *Applied Developmental Science, 9*, 174–187.

LeBuffe, P.A. (2002). *Can we foster resilience? An evaluation of a prevention program for preschoolers*. Conference proceedings of the 15th annual conference of a system of care for children's mental health: Expanding the research base.

LeBuffe, P.A. & Likins, L. (2001). Pilot study of the Devereux Early Childhood Assessment Program-Year 2. *Devereux early childhood initiative: Research bulletin #5*. Retrieved from http://www.devereux.org/site/PageServer?pagename=deci_research_bulletins

Leong, D. J. (2009). *Tools of the mind: Pre-K preschool*. Denver, CO: Metropolitan State College of Denver.

Lien-Thorne, S., & Kamps, D. (2005). Replication of the First Step to Success early intervention program. *Behavioral Disorders, 31*, 18–32.

Loeber, R., & Stouthamer-Loeber, M. (1998). Juvenile aggression at home and at school. In D. S. Elliott, K. R. Williams, & B. Hamburg (Eds.), *Violence in American schools* (pp. 94–126). Cambridge: Cambridge University Press.

Lucassen, P. L. B. J., Assendelft, W. J. J., Gubbles, J. W., van Eijk, J. T. M., van Geldrop, W., & Neven, A. K. (1998). Effectiveness of treatments for infantile colic: Systematic review. *British Medical Journal, 316*(7144), 1563–1569.

Lucassen, P. L. B. J., Assendelft, W. J. J., van Eijk, J. T. M., Gubbles, J. W., Douwes, A. C., & van Geldrop, W. J. (2001). Systematic review of the occurrence of infantile colic in the community. *Archives of Disease in Childhood, 84*(5), 398–403.

Luginbuehl, M., Bradley-Klug, K. L., Ferron, J., Anderson, W. M., & Benbadis, S. R. (2008). Pediatric sleep disorders: Validation of the sleep disorders inventory for students. *School Psychology Review, 37*(3), 409–431.

Lynch, K. B., Geller, S. R., & Schmidt, M. G. (2004). Multi-year evaluation of the effectiveness of a resilience-based prevention program for young children. *Journal of Primary Prevention, 24*(3), 335–353.

Lyons-Ruth, K., Zeanah, C. H., & Benoit, D. (2003). Disorder and risk for disorder during infancy and toddlerhood. In E. J. Mash & R. Barkley (Eds.), *Child psychopathology* (2nd ed.). New York: Guilford Press.

Maccoby, E. E., & Martin, J. A. (1983). Socialization in the context of the family: Parent–child interaction. In P. H. Mussen (Ed.) & E. M. Hetherington (Vol. Ed.), *Handbook of child psychology: Vol. 4. Socialization, personality, and social development* (4th ed., pp. 1–101). New York: Wiley.

Malott, R. W., & Suarez, E. A. (2004). *Principles of behavior* (5th ed.). Upper Saddle River, NJ: Prentice Hall.

Markie-Dadds, C., & Sanders, M. R. (2006a). A controlled evaluation of an enhanced self-directed behavioural family intervention for parents of children with conduct problems in rural and remote areas. *Behaviour Change, 23*(1), 55–72.

Markie-Dadds, C., & Sanders, M. R. (2006b). Self-directed Triple P (Positive Parenting Program) for mothers with children at-risk of developing conduct problems. *Behavioural and Cognitive Psychotherapy, 34*, 259–275.

Martin, A. J., & Sanders, M. R. (2003). Balancing work and family: A controlled evaluation of the Triple P- Positive Parenting Program as a work-site intervention. *Child and Adolescent Mental Health, 8*(4), 161–169.

Mathiesen, K. S., & Sanson, A. (2000). Dimensions of early childhood behavior problems: Stability and predictors of change from 18 to 30 months. *Journal of Abnormal Child Psychology, 28*, 15–31.

McConnell, S. R., McEvoy, M. A., & Priest, J. S. (2002). "Growing" measures for monitoring progress in early childhood education: A research and development process for Individual Growth and Development Indicators. *Assessment for Effective Intervention, 27*(4), 3–14.

McConnell, S. R., Priest, J. S., Davis, S., & McEvoy, M. A. (2002). Best practices in measuring growth and development in preschool children. In A. Thomas & J. Grimes (Eds.), *Best practices in school psychology IV* (4th ed., Vol. 2, pp. 1231–1246). Bethesda, MD: National Association of School Psychologists.

McGilly, K. (2000). *Chicago Born to Learn neuroscience project: Final report to Robert R. McCormick Tribune Foundation.* St. Louis, MO: Parents as Teachers National Center.

McIntyre, L. L. (2008). Parent training for young children with developmental disabilities: Randomized controlled trial. *American Journal on Mental Retardation, 113*(5), 356–368.

McMahon, R. J., & Forehand, R. L. (2003). *Helping the Noncompliant Child: Family-based treatment for oppositional behavior.* New York: Guilford.

McMahon, S. D., Washburn, J., Felix, E. D., Yakin, J., & Childrey, G. (2000). Violence prevention: Program effects on urban preschool and kindergarten children. *Applied and Preventive Psychology, 9*, 271–281.

Mendelsohn, A. L., Mogilner, L. N., Dreyer, B. P., Forman, J. A., Weinstein, S. C., Broderick, M., et al. (2001). The impact of a clinic-based literacy intervention on language development in inner-city preschool children. *Pediatrics, 107*(1), 130–134.

Mercy, J., & Saul, J. (2009). Creating a healthier future through early interventions for children. *Journal of the American Medical Association, 301*(21), 2262–2264.

Miller, L. S., Koplewicz, H. S., & Klein, R. G. (1997). Teacher ratings of hyperactivity, inattention, and conduct problems in preschoolers. *Journal of Abnormal Child Psychopathology, 25*(2), 113–119.

Mindell, J. A., Owens, J. A., & Carskadon, M. A. (1999). Developmental features of sleep. *Child and Adolescent Psychiatric Clinics of North America, 8*, 695–725.

Moore, B., & Beland, K. (1992). *Evaluation of Second Step: A violence prevention curriculum, preschool/kindergarten.* Seattle: Committee for Children.

National Association for the Education of Young Children (NAEYC). (1996). NAEYC position statement: Responding to linguistic and cultural diversity: Recommendations for effective early childhood education. *Young Children, 51*(4), 4–12.

National Center on Sexual Behavior of Youth (NCSBY). (2004). *Sexual development and sexual behavior problems in children ages 2-12* #4. Retrieved from http://www.ncsby.org/pages/publications/Sexual%20Devlopment%20of%20Children.pdf

National Center on Shaken Baby Syndrome. The period of purple crying. Retrieved February 1, 2013, from http://www.purplecrying.info/

National Research Council and Institute of Medicine. (2000). *From neurons to neighborhoods: The science of early childhood development.* Washington, DC: National Academy Press.

National Sleep Foundation. (2010). *Children and sleep.* Retrieved September 23, 2010, from http://www.sleepfoundation.org/article/sleep-topics/children-and-sleep

Neary, E. M., & Eyberg, S. M. (2002). Management of disruptive behavior in young children. *Infants and Young Children, 14,* 53–67.

Needleman, R. D. (2004). The preschool years. In R. E. Behrman, R. M. Kliegman, & H. B. Jenson (Eds.), *Nelson textbook of pediatrics* (17th ed., pp. 44–50). Philadelphia, PA: Elsevier Science.

Needleman, R., Toker, K. H., Dreyer, B. P., Klass, P., & Mendelsohn, A. L. (2005). Effectiveness of a primary care intervention to support reading aloud: A multicenter evaluation. *Ambulatory Pediatrics, 5*(4), 209–215.

Nevarez, M. D., Rifas-Shiman, S. L., Kleinman, K. P., Gillman, M. W., & Taveras, E. M. (2010). Associations of early life risk factors with infant sleep duration. *Academic Pediatrics, 10,* 187–193.

Newborg, J. (2005). *Battelle Developmental Inventory, Second Edition Screening Test.* Itasca, IL: Riverside Publishing.

Nixon, R. D. V., Sweeny, L., Erickson, D. B., & Touyz, S. W. (2003). Parent-child interaction therapy: A comparison of standard and abbreviated treatments for oppositional defiant preschoolers. *Journal of Consulting and Clinical Psychology, 71,* 251–260.

Olds, D. L., Eckenrode, J., Henderson, C. R., Kitzman, H., Powers, J., Cole, R., et al. (1997). Long-term effects of home visitation on maternal life course and child abuse and neglect: Fifteen-year follow-up of a randomized trial. *Journal of the American Medical Association, 278*(8), 637–643.

Olds, D. L., Henderson, C. R., Cole, R., Eckenrode, J., Kitzman, H., Luckey, D., et al. (1998). Long-term effects of nurse home visitation on children's criminal and antisocial behavior: Fifteen-year follow-up of a randomized controlled trial. *Journal of the American Medical Association, 280,* 1238–1244.

Olds, D. L., Henderson, C. R., & Kitzman, H. (1994). Does prenatal and infancy nurse home visitation have enduring effects on qualities of parental caregiving and child health at 25 to 50 months of life? *Pediatrics, 93*(1), 89–98.

Olds, D. L., Kitzman, H., Cole, R., Hanks, C. A., Arcoleo, K. J., Anson, E. A., et al. (2010). Enduring effects of prenatal and infancy home visiting by nurses on maternal life course and government spending. *Archives of Pediatric and Adolescent Medicine, 164*(5), 419–424.

Olds, D. L., Kitzman, H., Cole, R., Robinson, J., Sidora, K., Luckey, D. W., et al. (2004). Effects of nurse home visiting on maternal life course and child development: Age six follow-up results of a randomized trial. *Pediatrics, 114*(6), 1550–1559.

Olds, D. L., Kitzman, H., Hanks, C., Cole, R., Anson, E., Sidora-Arcoleo, K., et al. (2007). Effects of nurse home visiting on maternal and child functioning: Age nine follow-up of a randomized trial. *Pediatrics, 120,* 832–845.

Olds, D. L., Robinson, J., O'Brien, R., Luckey, D. W., Pettitt, L. M., Henderson, C. R., et al. (2002). Home visiting by paraprofessionals and by nurses: A randomized controlled trial. *Pediatrics, 110*(3), 486–496.

Olds, D. L., Robinson, J., Pettitt, L. M., Luckey, D. W., Holmberg, J., Ng, R. K., et al. (2004). Effects of home visits by paraprofessionals and be nurses: Age four follow-up results of a randomized trial. *Pediatrics, 114*(6), 1560–1568.

O'Neill, R. E., Horner, R. H., Albin, R. W., Sprague, J. R., Storey, K., & Newton, J. S. (1997). *Functional assessment and program development for problem behavior.* Pacific Grove, CA: Brooks/Cole Publishing.

Patterson, G. R. (1975). *A social learning approach to family intervention.* Eugene, OR: Castalia Publishing Company.

Patterson, G. R., DeBaryshe, B. D., & Ramsey, E. (1989). A developmental perspective on antisocial behavior. *American Psychologist, 44,* 329–335. (Reprinted from *Criminological theory: Past to present, essential readings,* 3rd ed., by R. Agnew & F. Cullen, Eds., 2006).

Pfannenstiel, J., & Seltzer, D. (1989). New parents as teachers: Evaluation of an early parent education program. *Early Childhood Research Quarterly, 4*, 1–18.

Powell, D., & Dunlap, G. (2009). Evidence-based social-emotional curricula and intervention packages for children 0–5 years and their families. (*Roadmap to Effective Intervention Practices*). Tampa, FL: University of South Florida, Technical Assistance Center on Social Emotional Intervention for Young Children.

Reid, M. J., & Webster-Stratton, C. (2001). The Incredible Years parent, teacher, and child intervention: Targeting multiple areas of risk for a young child with pervasive conduct problems using a flexible, manualized treatment program. *Cognitive and Behavioral Practice, 8*, 377–386.

Reid, M. J., Webster-Stratton, C., & Beauchaine, T. P. (2002). Parent training in Head Start: A comparison of program response among African American, Asian American, Caucasian, and Hispanic mothers. *Prevention Science, 2*(4), 209–227.

Rickel, A. U., & Burgio, J. C. (1982). Assessing social competence in lower income preschool children. *American Journal of Community Psychology, 10*, 149–153.

Roberts, M. (2012). Parents' Evaluation of Developmental Status. *In the Fourteenth Mental Measurements Yearbook*. Retrieved from EBSCO Mental Measurements Yearbook database.

Roberts, C., Mazzucchelli, T., Studman, L., & Sanders, M. R. (2006). A randomized control trial of behavioral family intervention for young children with developmental and behavioral problems. *Journal of Clinical Child and Adolescent Psychology, 35*(2), 180–193.

Robins, D. L., Fein, D., & Barton, M. (1999). *The Modified Checklist for Autism in Toddlers*. Retrieved from http://www2.gsu.edu/~wwwpsy/faculty/robins.htm (Self-published).

Russell Carter, D., & Horner, R. H. (2007). Adding functional behavioral assessment to First Step to Success: A case study. *Journal of Positive Behavior Interventions, 9*, 229–238.

Sackett, D. L., Rosenberg, W., Gray, J. A., Haynes, R., & Richardson, W. S. (1996). Evidence-based medicine: What it is and what it isn't. *British Medical Journal, 312*, 71–72.

Salinas, A., Smith, J. C., & Armstrong, K. (2011). Engaging fathers in behavioral parent training: Listening to father' voices. *Journal of Pediatric Nursing, 26*(4), 3–8.

Sallows, G. O., & Graupner, T. D. (2005). Intensive behavioral treatment for children with autism: Four-year outcome and predictors. *American Journal on Mental Retardation, 110*(6), 417–438.

Sampers, J., Anderson, K. G., Hartung, C. M., & Scambler, D. J. (2001). Parent training programs for young children with behavior problems. *Infant-Toddler Intervention, 11*(2), 91–110.

Sanders, M. R., Cann, W., & Markie-Dadds, C. (2003). The Triple P- Positive Parenting Program: A universal population-level approach to the prevention of child abuse. *Child Abuse Review, 12*(3), 155–171.

Sanders, L. M., Gershon, T. D., Huffman, L. C., & Mendoza, F. S. (2000). Prescribing books for immigrant children. *Archives of Pediatrics & Adolescent Medicine, 154*, 771–777.

Sanders, M. R., Markie-Dadds, C., Tully, L., & Bor, W. (2000). The Triple P- Positive Parenting Program: A comparison of enhanced, standard, and self directed behavioral family intervention for parents of children with early onset conduct problems. *Journal of Consulting and Clinical Psychology, 68*(4), 624–640.

Sanders, M. R., Montgomery, D., & Brechman-Toussaint, M. (2000). The mass media and the prevention of child behavior problems: The evaluation of a television series to promote positive outcomes for parents and their children. *Journal of Child Psychology and Psychiatry, 41*(7), 939–948.

Sanders, M. R., Pidgeon, A., Gravestock, F., Connors, M. D., Brown, S., & Young, R. M. (2004). Does parental attributional retraining and anger management enhance the effects of the Triple P- Positive Parenting Program with parents at-risk of child maltreatment? *Behavior Therapy, 35*(3), 513–535.

Schopler, E., Reichler, R. J., & Renner, B. R. (1988). *Childhood Autism Rating Scale*. Los Angeles, CA: Western Psychological Resources.

Schuhmann, E. M., Foote, R., Eyberg, S. M., Boggs, S., & Algina, J. (1998). Parent-child interaction therapy: Interim report of a randomized trial with short-term maintenance. *Journal of Clinical Child Psychology, 27*, 34–45.

Schum, T. R., Kolb, T. M., McAuliffe, T. L., Simms, M., Underhill, R., & Lewis, M. (2002). The sequential acquisition of toilet training skills: A descriptive study of gender and age differences in normal children. *Pediatrics, 109*(e3), e48.

Serna, L. A., Forness, S. R., & Mattern, N. (2002, November). *Relationship between improvement in psychiatric symptoms and improvement in functional impairment: Data from a primary prevention program in a Head Start classroom*. Paper presented at the annual TECBD Conference on Severe Behavior Disorders of Children and Youth, Tempe, Arizona.

Serna, L. A., Nielsen, M. E., Lambros, K., & Forness, S. R. (2000). Primary prevention with children at risk for emotional and behavioral disorders: Data on a universal intervention for Head Start classrooms. *Behavioral Disorders, 26*, 70–84.

Serna, L. A., Nielsen, M. E., Mattern, N., & Forness, S. R. (2003). Primary mental health prevention in Head Start classrooms: Partial replication with teachers as intervenors. *Behavioral Disorders, 28*, 124–129.

Sharif, I., Rieber, S., & Ozuah, P. O. (2002). Exposure to reach out and red and vocabulary outcomes in inner city preschoolers. *Journal of the National Medical Association, 94*(3), 171–177.

Shure, M. B., & Spivack, G. (1979). Interpersonal cognitive problem solving and primary prevention: Programming for preschool and kindergarten children. *Journal of Clinical Child Psychology, 2*, 89–94.

Shure, M. B., & Spivack, G. (1980). Interpersonal problem solving as a mediator of personal adjustment in preschool and kindergarten children. *Journal of Applied Developmental Psychology, 1*, 29–44.

Shure, M. B., & Spivack, G. (1982). Interpersonal problem solving in young children: A cognitive approach to prevention. *American Journal of Community Psychology, 10*(3), 341–356.

Silverstein, M., Iverson, L., & Lozano, P. (2002). An English-language clinic-based literacy program is effective for a multilingual population. *Pediatrics, 109*(5), 1–6.

Simpson, R. L. (2005). Evidence-based practices and students with autism spectrum disorders. *Focus on Autism and Other Developmental Disabilities, 20*(3), 140–149.

Smith, T., Groen, A. D., & Wynn, J. W. (2000). Randomized trial of intensive early intervention for children with pervasive developmental disorder. *American Journal on Mental Retardation, 105*(4), 269–285.

Smyke, A. T., Dumitrescu, A., & Zeanah, C. H. (2002). Attachment disturbances in young children: The continuum of caretaking casualty. *Journal of the American Academy of Child and Adolescent Psychiatry, 41*, 972–982.

Society for Research in Child Development. (2009). *Healthy development: A Summit on Young Children's Mental Health. Partnering with communication scientists, collaborating across disciplines, and leveraging impact to promote Children's Mental Health*. Washington, DC: Society for Research in Child Development.

Spencer, P. (2000). *Parenting: Guide to your toddler*. New York: Ballantine Books.

Squires, J., Bricker, D., Twombly, F., & Yockelson, M. S. (2001). *Ages and stages questionnaire: Social emotional (ASQ: SE): A parent completed child monitoring system*. Baltimore: Paul H. Brookes Publishing.

St. James-Roberts, I., & Halil, A. T. (1991). Infant crying patterns in the first year: Normal community and clinical findings. *Journal of Child Psychology and Psychiatry, 32*, 951–968.

Strain, P. S. (1987). Parent training with young autistic children: A report on the LEAP model. *Zero to Three, 7*(3), 7–12.

Strain, P. S., & Cordisco, L. (1993). The LEAP preschool model: Description and outcomes. In S. Harris & J. Handleman (Eds.), *Preschool education programs for children with autism* (pp. 224–244). Austin, TX: PRO-ED.

Strain, P. S., Kohler, F. W., & Goldstein, H. (1996). Learning experiences…An alternative program: Peer-mediated interventions for young children with autism. In E. D. Hibbs & P. S. Jensen (Eds.), *Psychosocial treatments from child and adolescent disorders: Empirically based strategies for clinical practice*. Washington, DC: American Psychological Association.

Sugai, G., & Horner, R. H. (2005). School-wide positive behavior supports: Achieving and sustaining effective learning environments for all students. In W. H. Heward (Ed.), *Focus on behavior analysis in education: Achievements, challenges, and opportunities* (pp. 90–102). Upper Saddle River, NJ: Pearson Prentice-Hall.

Taylor, C. A., Manganello, J. A., Lee, S. J., & Rice, J. C. (2010). Mothers' spanking of 3-year-old children and subsequent risk of children's aggressive behavior. *Pediatrics, 125*(5), 1049–1050.

Taylor, T. K., Webster-Stratton, C., Feil, E. G., Broadbent, B., Widdop, C. S., & Severson, H. H. (2008). Computer-based intervention with coaching: An example using the Incredible Years program. *Cognitive Behavior Therapy, 37*(4), 233–246.

Theriot, J. A., Franco, S. M., Sisson, B. A., Metcalf, S. C., Kennedy, M. A., & Bada, H. S. (2003). The impact of early literacy guidance on language skills of 3-year-olds. *Clinical Pediatrics, 42*, 165–172.

Tremblay, R. E. (2000). The development of aggressive behavior during childhood: What have we learned in the past century? *International Journal of Behavioral Development, 24*(2), 129–141.

Turner, K. M. T., & Sanders, M. R. (2006). Help when it's needed first: A controlled evaluation of brief, preventive behavioral family intervention in a primary care setting. *Behavior Therapy, 37*(2), 131–142.

Turner, K. M. T., Sanders, M. R., & Wall, C. R. (1994). Behavioural parent training versus dietary education in the treatment of children with persistent feeding difficulties. *Behaviour Change, 11*(4), 242–258.

U.S. Department of Health and Human Services. (2010). *Addressing the needs of young children and their families.* Retrieved February 12, 2013, from http://store.samhsa.gov/product/Addressing-the-Mental-Health-Needs-of-Young-Children-and-Their-Families/SMA10-4547

U.S. Public Health Service. (2001). *Report of the surgeon general on Children's Mental Health.* Rockville, MD: Author.

Vacca, J. J. (2005). Review of ages & stages questionnaires: Social-emotional: A parent-completed, child-monitoring system for social emotional behaviors. *In the Sixteenth Mental Measurements Yearbook.* Retrieved from EBSCO Mental Measurements Yearbook database.

Vacca, J. (2012). Review of ages & stages questionnaires: Social-emotional: A parent-completed, child-monitoring system for social-emotional behaviors. *In the Sixteenth Mental Measurements Yearbook.* Retrieved from EBSCO Mental Measurements Yearbook database.

Van Der Heyden, A. M., & Snyder, P. (2006). Integrating frameworks from early childhood intervention and school psychology to accelerate growth for all young children. *School Psychology Review, 35*(4), 519–534.

Van Haneghan, J. P. (2009). Validating assessment for learning: Consequential and systems approach. *Journal of Multidisciplinary Evaluation, 6*, 23–31.

Vismara, L. A., & Rogers, S. J. (2008). The Early Start Denver Model: A case study of an innovative practice. *Journal of Early Intervention, 31*(1), 91–108.

Vygotsky, L. S. (1978). *Mind in Society: The development of higher psychological processes.* Cambridge: Harvard University Press.

Wackerle, A. K. (2007). *Test review: Early childhood research institute on measuring growth and development. (1998). Selection of general growth outcomes for children between birth and age eight* (Tech. Rep. No. 2). Minneapolis, MN: Center for early education and development. Reviewed by Alisha K. Wackerle. *Assessment for Effective Intervention, 33*, 51–54.

Wagner, M. & Spiker, D. (2001). *Multisite Parents as Teachers evaluation: Experience and outcomes for children and families.* Menlo Park, CA: SRI International. Retrieved from http://policyweb.sri.com/cehs/publications/patfinal.pdf

Walker, D., Cartta, J. J., Greenwood, C. R., & Buzhardt, J. (2008). The use of individual growth and developmental indicators for progress monitoring and intervention decision making in early education. *Exceptionality, 16*, 33–47.

Walker, H. M., Severson, H. H., Feil, E. G., Stiller, B., & Golly, A. (1998). First step to success: Intervening at the point of school entry to prevent antisocial behavior patterns. *Psychology in the Schools, 35*(3), 259–269.

Webster-Stratton, C., & Hammond, M. (1988). Maternal depression and its relationship to life stress, perceptions of child behavior problems, parenting behaviors, and child conduct problems. *Journal of Abnormal Child Psychology, 16*(3), 299–315.

Webster-Stratton, C., & Hammond, M. (1997). Treating children with early-onset conduct problems: A comparison of child and parent training interventions. *Journal of Consulting and Clinical Psychology, 65*, 93–109.

Webster-Stratton, C., & Reid, M. J. (1999, November). *Treating children with early-onset conduct problems: The importance of teacher training.* Paper presented at the meeting of the Association for Advancement of Behavior Therapy, Toronto, Canada.

Webster-Stratton, C., & Reid, M. J. (2003). The Incredible Years parents, teachers, and children training series. In A. E. Kazdin & J. R. Weisz (Eds.), *Evidence-based psychotherapies for children and adolescents.* New York: Guilford.

Webster-Stratton, C., Reid, M. J., & Hammond, M. (2001a). Preventing conduct problems, promoting social competence: A parent and teacher training partnership in Head Start. *Journal of Clinical Child Psychology, 30*, 283–302.

Webster-Stratton, C., Reid, M. J., & Hammond, M. (2001b). Social skills and problem solving training for children with early-onset conduct problems: Who benefits? *Journal of Child Psychology and Psychiatry, 42*, 943–952.

Weinberg, K. M., & Tronick, E. Z. (1997). Maternal depression and infant maladjustment: A failure of mutual regulation. In J. Noshpitz (Ed.), *The handbook of child and adolescent psychiatry.* New York: Wiley.

Weitzman, C. C., Roy, L., Walls, T., & Tomlin, R. (2004). More evidence for Reach Out and Read: A home-based study. *Pediatrics, 113*(5), 1248–1253.

Wells, K. C. (2003). Adaptations for specific populations. In R. J. McMahon & R. L. Forehand (Eds.). Helping the Noncompliant Child: Family-based Treatment for Oppositional Behavior (pp. 182–200). New York: Guilford.

Wells, K. C., & Egan, J. (1988). Social learning and systems family therapy for childhood oppositional disorder: Comparative treatment outcome. *Comprehensive Psychiatry, 29*, 138–146.

Wetherby, A., & Prizant, B. (2002). *Communication and symbolic behavior scales developmental profile-first normed edition.* Baltimore: Paul H. Brookes.

Williams, J. L. (2007). Caregivers' Perceptions of the Effectiveness of the *Helping Our Toddlers, Developing Our Children's Skills* Parent Training Program: A Pilot Study. *Psychological and Social Foundations.* Tampa: University of South Florida. Educational Specialist (EdS): 163.

Williams, J. L. (2009). *Helping Our Toddlers, Developing Our Children's Skills (HOT DOCS):* An Investigation of a Parenting Program to Address Challenging Behavior in Young Children. *Psychological and Social Foundations.* Tampa: University of South Florida. Doctorate of Philosophy (PhD): 217.

Williams, J., Agazzi, H., & Armstrong, K. (2011). Evaluating outcomes of a behavioral parent training program for caregivers of young children: Waitlist control versus immediate treatment. *Journal of Early Childhood and Infant Psychology, 7*, 26–45.

Williams, J., Armstrong, K., Agazzi, H., & Bradley-Klug, K. (2010). Helping Our Toddlers, Developing Our Children's Skills (HOT DOCS): A parenting intervention to prevent and address challenging behavior in young children. *Journal of Early Childhood and Infant Psychology, 6*, 1–20.

Williams, J., Klinepeber, K., & Palmes, G. (2004). Diagnosis and treatment of behavioral health disorders in pediatric practice. *Pediatrics, 114*, 601–606.

Wright Carroll, D. (2009). Toward multiculturalism competence: A practical model for implementation in the schools. In J. M. Jones (Ed.), *The Psychology of Multiculturalism in the Schools: A primer for training, practice, and research.* Bethesda: National Association of School Psychologists.

Wyman, P. A., Cowen, E. L., Work, W. C., Hoyt-Meyers, L. A., Magnus, K. B., & Fagen, D. B. (1999). Caregiving and developmental factors differentiating young at-risk urban children showing resilient versus stress-affected outcomes: A replication and extension. *Child Development, 709*, 645–659.

Young, K. T., Davis, K., Schoen, C., & Parker, S. (1998). Listening to parents. A national survey of parents with young children. *Archives of Pediatrics Adolescent Medicine, 152*(3), 255–262.

Zigler, E., Pfannenstiel, J. C., & Seitz, V. (2008). The Parents as Teachers program and school success: A replication and extension. *Journal of Primary Prevention, 29*, 103–120.

Zisser, A., & Eyberg, S.M. Parent-child interaction therapy and the treatment of disruptive behavior disorders. In J.R. Weisz & A.E. Kazdin (Eds.) *Evidence-based psychotherapies for children and adolescents* (2nd ed., pp. 179–193). New York: Guilford Press.

Zubrick, S. R., Northey, K., Silburn, S. R., Lawrence, D., Williams, A. A., Blair, E., et al. (2005). Prevention of child behavior problems through universal implementation of a group behavioral family intervention. *Prevention Science, 6*(4), 287–304.

Zuckerman, B. (2009). Promoting early literacy in pediatric practice: Twenty years of reach out and read. *Pediatrics, 124*, 1660–1665.

About the Authors

Kathleen Hague Armstrong, Ph.D., NCSP, is a professor of Pediatrics at the University of South Florida College of Medicine, licensed psychologist and Past-President of Florida Association of Infant Mental Health. She has extensive experience working with young children and families with behavioral issues, graduate teaching, and has authored several articles and book chapters on early childhood topics and parenting.

Julia A. Ogg, Ph.D., NCSP, is an assistant professor in the School Psychology Program at the University of South Florida and is trained in recognized evidence-based programs including *The Incredible Years* and *Parent Child Interaction Therapy*.

Ashley N. Sundman-Wheat, Ph.D., NCSP, is a practicing school psychologist for Pasco County Schools, FL. She has extensive work experiences in early childhood settings, such as Head Start, and the Early Steps program.

Audra St. John Walsh, Ph.D., NCSP, is a school psychologist working in Pinellas County Schools, FL and the University of South Florida Pediatric Special Immunology Program. She has a strong background in early intervention from her years of working with families as an Infant Toddler Developmental Specialist.

K.H. Armstrong et al., *Evidence-Based Interventions for Children with Challenging Behavior*, DOI 10.1007/978-1-4614-7807-2, © Springer Science+Business Media New York 2014

Index

K.H. Armstrong et al., *Evidence-Based Interventions for Children
with Challenging Behavior*, DOI 10.1007/978-1-4614-7807-2,
© Springer Science+Business Media New York 2014

Printed by Publishers' Graphics LLC